Aging in the Designed Environment

Aging in the Designed Environment

Margaret A. Christenson
Principle Author

Ellen D. Taira
Editor

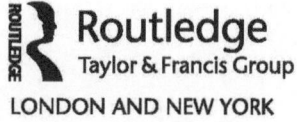
Routledge
Taylor & Francis Group

LONDON AND NEW YORK

First published 1990 by The Haworth Press, Inc.

2 Park Square, Milton Park, Abingdon, Oxon OX14 4RN
711 Third Avenue, New York, NY 10017, USA

Routledge is an imprint of the Taylor & Francis Group, an informa business

Aging in the Designed Environment has also been published as *Physical & Occupational Therapy in Geriatrics*, Volume 8, Numbers 3/4 1990.

First issued in paperback 2016

Copyright © 1990 Taylor& Francis.

Library of Congress Cataloging-in-Publication Data

Christenson, Margaret A.
Aging in the designed environment / Margaret A. Christenson : Ellen D. Taira, editor.
    p. cm.
    Published also as Physical & occupational therapy in geriatrics, vol. 8, no. 3/4, 1990.
    Includes bibliographical references.
    1. Long-term care facilities — Design and construction. 2. Nursing homes — Design and construction. 3. Aged — Long term care. I. Taira, Ellen D. II. Title
RA998.5.C48   1990
725'.56 — dc20   90-4421
                                         CIP

ISBN 13: 978-1-560-24031-0 (hbk)
ISBN 13: 978-1-138-96635-2 (pbk)

Aging in the Designed Environment

CONTENTS

ABOUT THE AUTHOR

Margaret A. Christenson, MPH, OTR, geriatric environmental consultant, is President and Founder of Geriatric Environmental Concepts, Inc. She is also Teaching Specialist of designed environments and aging at the University of Minnesota. In 1989, Ms. Christenson was awarded the Minnesota Occupational Therapist of the Year for her efforts to maximize the functional abilities of the elderly through environmental modifications. As a frequent lecturer and seminar leader, she has spoken on age-related sensory changes and understanding psychological components of the designed environment. She is also an active consultant to architects and developers of residential housing and long-term care facilities.

Ms. Christenson has published several articles and a book focusing on age-related adaptions in the elderly environment. She is a member of the American Occupational Therapy Association and the American Society on Aging, and she has served on the Forum on Technology and Aging for that organization. She is also an active member of the Minnesota Gerontological Society and has chaired a focus group on "Technology and Aging in Minnesota."

Preface

"... Fearfully and wonderfully made."

—Psalm 139:14b

When we gaze at a new born or observe the skills of a young athlete, we exclaim concerning the potential and intricacies of the human body. As a person ages we are less prone to consider with amazement this creation. When we consider how well most older persons do function with the limitations that age presents, we begin to realize that the potential for the elderly is still vast and, if placed in the properly designed environment, their capabilities can be maximized.

The environment is too often not designed to consider the limited capacity of the older person. This publication focuses on interventions in the designed environment of the home, senior housing project and long term care facility that will compensate for age-related changes.

Margaret A. Christenson, MPH, OTR

Introduction

This book, devoted exclusively to the topic of aging and environmental design, is the culmination of many years of thinking, planning, reading, writing and researching by gerontologist/occupational therapist Margaret Christenson, who has been a pioneer in a specialized field bridging at least three areas: rehabilitation, design and aging. Using her many years of interest in design, her thirty plus years as an occupational therapist and her concern for the needs of the older person, Margaret Christenson has formed a consultation firm, Geriatric Environmental Concepts, Inc. to deal with these issues. Those of us who have been frustrated by the lack of environmental solutions to the problems encountered in the long term care setting especially welcome her common sense solutions that combine technical expertise, medical knowledge and a keen desire to assist older persons to "age in place."

Every therapist providing rehabilitation services to the elderly has met more than a few clients/residents whose disability should not have happened. Ms. Christenson covers the standard loose carpets and poor lighting problems that contribute to falls as well as labeling other every day occurrences such as carpet patterns and window glare that are not uncommon, yet not frequent enough to become an aggregated problem. What Aging in the Designed Environment does so well is to describe small solutions to potentially large problems. For example, well placed art work that can consistently direct a disoriented person to their room and may reduce the need for constant redirection by staff.

Aging in the Designed Environment is a fitting contribution to a decade of emerging importance for environmental adaptations in long term care. This book makes it possible for geriatric rehabilitation specialists to consider the physical sensory and cognitive changes that are a normal part of aging as they are impacted by the residential and institutional environment of the older person.

Ellen Taira,
Editor
Physical & Occupational Therapy in Geriatrics

Adaptations of the Physical Environment to Compensate for Sensory Changes

INTRODUCTION

The physical environment, as it relates to the dependencies of older adults, remains one of the most overlooked areas in environmental design. In order to move beyond this status quo, persons responsible for planning that environment must develop a new understanding of ways in which their influence can improve the older adult's physical and mental functioning. This section deals with age-related changes in vision, hearing, taste, smell, touch and kinesthetic systems, and provides recommendations for environmental adaptation and modifications which may compensate for the changes in each of these systems.

As people age, certain sensory changes cause them to perceive and respond to the physical environment in different ways: a person may walk more slowly, move more deliberately, hold reading material farther from the eyes, or strain to distinguish a voice in a crowd. As more and more limitations in functioning are experienced, the person becomes more dependent on that environment for support. Indeed, "as strength fails and as the sensory organs incur deprivations, the individual experiencing these losses reaches out to both the general social environment and the physical environment in order to continue functioning (Koncelik, 1976, pg. 15)."

Sensory changes not only increase as people grow older but are usually compounded by the simultaneous occurrence of changes in several sensory systems. However, the age of onset and the rate of decline for these functions differ markedly among and within the various sensory systems (Corso, 1971).

Age-related changes occur gradually, and most people continue to function adequately at home or in familiar surroundings. Yet, for a growing number of persons, sensory changes are so altered that functioning in the environment is difficult at best and may even be impossible. The impact sensory changes have on the person with confusion must be considered when planning environments for those individuals with dementia. The reduced sensory acuity that accompanies age produces sensory deprivation.

When an older person does not respond to "normal" amounts of stimulation, increased stimulus is required. However, too many changes may result in sensory distortion. With impaired hearing, for instance, usually the higher ranges of tones are affected. But, when volume is increased to hear these tones, even fuzzily, the volume may be too loud in the low ranges where hearing is relatively normal. Thus deprivation, distortion, and overload may exist simultaneously for the older person (Wolanin & Phillips, 1981).

Although sensory alteration may arise in any setting, the institutionalized elderly are particularly vulnerable. In addition to experiencing greater impairment, these adults also face increased exposure to situations offering little variety or stimulation.

Sensory deprivation research suggests "that most impairments are confined to the 'visual modality' and include a general decrease in the efficiency of perception of stimuli (Schultz, 1965, pg. 97)." Parent (1978), has summarized the effects of sensory deprivation to include: loss of the ability to concentrate, disorientation and reported hallucinations, and delusions. Illusions are also common. In early studies done in the Hebb's Laboratory at McGill University, lack of sensory stimulation created significant changes in the individuals under study. Bexton's early research (1954) brought to light the dependency individuals have upon the environment.

The recent increase in the development of special long-term care units designed for those with senile dementia, requires that we attempt to perceive the environment from the perspective of residents. Since the person with dementia will also be experiencing the normal age-related sensory changes, adapting the physical environment to meet the needs of the confused person becomes even more critical. New findings concerning the behavior of the person with dementia must be applied to the less structured institutional situations, as well as the more conventional long-term care unit.

The environment should be constructed so that it enhances the functioning of all persons with sensory deficits. Designing and decorating should provide "redundant" cuing. The combined input of hearing the sound of kitchen activities, smelling the aroma of food cooking, and seeing and touching the table and dishes tells us, through redundant cuing, "This is the dining room" (Pastalan, 1973). Provision of such multiple input allows older persons to compensate for losses by using the best combination of remaining sensitivities rather than being dependent on only one sense.

Those who provide care to older adults must be aware however of the possible negative effects of redundant cuing. For example, if a confused person is seated at the table long before meal time, the redundant input implies eating and the person may react by simply becoming more agitated.

Landmarks or prominent features marking a particular locality can help an older person be oriented in a space. Just as certain buildings, and monuments serve as focal points in a city, picture groupings or special textured objects or surfaces can be used as landmarks in an older person's environment. These landmarks give cues concerning where to sit, to turn or to stop. Those who work with older adults should help them understand the cues by explaining their purpose and by using the cues to orient them. For example: One might say to the person in the nursing home, "This is your room, Mr. Smith, here by the large picture of red flowers." For the person living at home the verbal cue might be, "Ellen, we're back at your house, here's your mailbox with the red cardinal on it."

Lawton (1980) has classified environments on the basis of demand character. Some environments make greater behavioral demands on people than others. This dimension is called "environmental press," following the terminology of psychologist Henry Murray. It specifies that those with higher levels of competence can adapt to a wider range of environmental press with greater likelihood of experiencing favorable adaptive outcomes.

The environment has the greatest effect on the person with the least capability. Although slight increases in environmental press may result in maladaptive behavior, other small changes such as increased lighting, reduced noise, or added texture may cause meaningful improvement in behavior (Kiernat, 1985). It is also thought that human interaction with the environment and its objects has a major role in eliciting intelligent behavior. Many researchers contend that coping with appropriate environmental complexity contributes to mental function.

Designing an environment with these changes in mind creates a supportive environment that makes it possible for more individuals to function at their maximum capabilities. In addition, most adaptations will facilitate functioning for formal and informal caregivers as well.

VISUAL ADAPTATION

For the older person with visual problems, the environment needs to be more structured and predictable, as well as visually richer (Wolanin & Phillips, 1981). Snyder et al. (1976), in a study of 295 extended care residents over 65 years of age, found that 24 percent were legally blind (20/200 with correction) and 35 percent had low visual acuity (20/70 to 20/100 with correction). Since many of these conditions were unknown prior to the study, many corrective measures were consequently initiated. Visual screening should be done initially as well as periodically to determine any resulting change in the older person's level of need. Hiatt (1980) has reported a thorough visual screening procedure that can be administered in the nursing home as well as other settings. This procedure includes testing for: near vision, far vision, mobility, fear and security, sensitivities and special implications of specific eye conditions. A practical guide for caring for the visually impaired older person is available from any local Society for the Blind.

As an individual ages, structural changes occur in the eyes that affect vision. Some of these changes involve the lens, which shows a gradual increase of tissue at the center. In the internal structures of the eyeball, small opacities and vascularites develop. These alterations are further complicated by changes in the surrounding eye muscles and decreased elasticity of the lens. These changes cause a scattering of light that blurs the retinal image (Corso, 1971), decreasing an individual's ability to see objects clearly and increasing the susceptibility to glare.

Visual Aids

Large contrasting lettering on signs and on written directions will facilitate vision for the person with acuity problems. Letters for signs should be a minimum of 5/8 inch in height and recessed or raised 1/32 inch for readability through touch (Bowersox, 1979). Lettering on signs also should contrast with the background (USAF, 1984). Large white or light colored letters, on a black or dark colored background will help older adults distinguish those letters from the surrounding background (Reznikoff, 1979). In the institutional setting, any type of name tag should also have large lettering, since typed lettering is too small for the older adult to read easily. A large-print calendar in a corridor can function both as landmark and an orienting aid. Clock faces with large light numbers on dark non-reflectant background should be located at the older person's level.

The ability of the eye to differentiate detail is regulated by the process of accommodation and is dependent on the elasticity of the eye. Presbyopia, an age-related difficulty of accommodation, is a loss of the len's elasticity and thus the ability of the ciliary muscle to affect the curvature of the lens (Corso, 1971). This leads to decreased focusing on the detail of objects close at hand or at varied distances. For example, the older person who is playing cards will require more time than a younger person to shift the focus of vision from cards held in the hand to cards placed in the middle of the table.

In the initial stages of presbyopia, corrective lenses for near vision will rectify the difficulty of reading fine print close at hand. But correction may not be possible in later stages. At that point, books and periodicals with larger print and greater intensity, and contrast offer the older person the most benefit. Low vision aids such as magnifying glasses, preferably lighted, should be made available.

In a case study (Kornzweig, 1976) done at the Jewish-Home and Hospital for the Aged in New York, to determine if low-vision aids would be used by a group of visually impaired elderly, the following results were noted: Of the 83 residents examined initially, 62 were helped, to a greater or lesser degree by using the aids. Some of the low-vision aids utilized included: large-print reading material, playing cards, bingo cards, and telephone dials.

Many items useful to low-vision persons are available through the American Foundation for the Blind (Cristarella, 1976). These devises include specially adapted watches and clocks. The partially sighted can also benefit from self-care techniques used by the blind. One such technique involves leaving in place commonly used items and arranging food and utensils in the same places for every meal.

Lighting

As the lens of the eye becomes less transparent and thickens, there is an increase in the amount of light required for a person to be able to see (Corso, 1971). Pastalan (1976) developed an empathic model that determined that a person of 80 years of age needs approximately three times more light to read than the person 15-20 years of age. As the transparency of the lens decreases and becomes more opaque, a cataract forms. By the time a person reaches 70 years of age, some evidence of cataract formation is the rule, rather than the exception (Colavita, 1978). The amount of light that reaches the retina of the eye is also reduced by the size of the pupil, which becomes smaller as the individual ages. Only about one third of the light that arrives at the retina of a 20-year-old falls on the retina of a 60-year-old (Corso, 1971). In addition, the ability to function in low light also decreases.

Reading and close work can be aided by increased illumination with task lighting, such as floor or table lamps with three-way bulbs. These allow better direction and level of lighting than conventional overhead fixtures (Bowersox, 1978). However, bulbs should not be exposed or installed directly in the older person's line of vision since this creates direct glare.

Glare is a painful overload problem caused by too much illumination. Sensitivity to glare is caused by the opacity of the lens, as well as changes within the eyeball. Glare problems may develop from both a direct or indirect source. Direct glare occurs when light reaches the eye directly from its source. Indirect glare arises when the light reflects into the eye rebounding off another surface (Birren, 1977).

Examples of such glare would include: Sunlight reflecting off a highly polished floor or stainless steel appliances walkers, plastic-covered furniture, and waxed floors. Even dishes and silverware can reflect an uncomfortable level of light (Wolanin, 1981; Hiatt, 1979; Bowersox, 1978; Koncelik, 1976).

To reduce glare, avoid using glossy paint and shiny laminated plastic table tops. Windows may be covered with glare-reducing film, tinted mylar shades, mini-blinds or pleated polyester window shades. If the older adult suffers from incontinence, velour-like plastics or polyester upholstery using a vapor barrier can be used to decrease odors. This upholstery is installed with velcro and can be laundered in a clothes washer and line dried. This special fabric provides the texture and warmth of upholstery while still addressing the problems of maintenance.

When preparing publicity for seniors use the dull side of poster board to make signs and posters. Lobby directions and other glass-covered surfaces should have non-glare glass. Light reflected from structures or surfaces outside a window, water from a pond or lake, a white wall, can also cause glare.

Outdoor seating areas should be provided with sun screens, such as gazebos, wood trellises and fences. Roof overhangs, awnings, or building recesses also limit direct sunlight penetration. To reduce glare, consideration should be given to the location and types of trees used to shade courtyards and major glass areas. Older persons select glare-free areas where they can sit where people are likely to pass (Regnier & Pynoos, 1987).

Wall-mounted valance or cove lighting that conceals the source of light, and then spreads it indirectly upon the ceiling and down on the floor is recommended to eliminate glare. Better lighting will make it easier for older persons to recognize faces and improve communications. A study by Snyder (1978), showed that increased accidents in a nursing home seemed to be directly related to energy conservationists who turned out every other light in the hall, causing the contrast between bright and shadowed areas of the hallways to appear as steps, particularly to people with perceptual difficulties.

Fluorescent fixtures can reduce glare, but they must be selected carefully and ballasts checked regularly to be sure flickering is minimized (Bowersox, 1978). "Fluorescent light flickers which eludes many younger persons is quite evident to older people, causing tearing, headaches and general unattentiveness. Exposed lamp fixtures and improperly functioning ballasts may be causes" (Hiatt, 1979, pg. 8).

Fluorescent lighting should be combined with incandescent lighting in areas where extensive lighting is needed, e.g., bathrooms, reading areas, and so on. Whenever fluorescent light sources are used, choose warm-white deluxe or prime color tubes. Paraboloid patterned fixture covers on fluorescent lights, which are made of anodized aluminum and are often used in libraries, provide better light distribution and eliminate glare.

Fluorescent lighting has been eliminated from some long-term care units designed for terminal patients because of the flickering that can occur (Peppard, 1984).

Glare has other effects. Snyder (1978) reports that the attention span may be increased when reflection is reduced. Furthermore, bright lights and glare may distract older persons, especially those who have difficulty concentrating.

In some states rules and regulations for long-term care facilities defining the interior design, run counter to what researchers have discovered about the aging process. Many states, for example, require placing ceiling lights in the middle of every resident room. Such a situation creates direct glare for the person who is lying down, and residents who are sitting express a preference for focused task lighting such as table and or desk lamps. Translucent wall or post fixtures, placed at eye level cause direct glare and should not be used.

Sight recovery for the older person is delayed when moving from a light area to a dark or darker area. Moving into a much lighter area also creates problems. For an older person, turning on a light in a dark room can produce the same effect that one experiences when a flashbulb flashes (Hatton, 1977). When older persons must come from a light area to a darker area, such as into a foyer or into their own room from a hall, no furniture or other objects should be placed by the door. Adequate time should also be allowed for proper sight recovery (Pastalan, 1976). In addition, night lights should be installed in and on the way to the bathroom. A switch placed outside the bathroom, with a light built into the switch plate as a night light, can also be very helpful. Finally, lighting within the entire living environment or facility should be as consistent as possible.

Color Perception

With increasing age, the lens of the eye takes on a yellowish color which alters the quality of light entering the pupil. This gradual yellowing impairs the perception of certain colors, particularly greens, blues, and purples. Dark shades of navy, brown, and black are probably not distinguishable except under the most intense lighting conditions. Furthermore, differences between pastel colors such as blues, beiges, yellows and pinks are often impossible to detect. "This is why many older people will not see their room as being distinct from their neighbor's" (Hiatt, 1979, pg. 9).

One study indicated a preference on the part of older persons for primary, secondary, or tertiary colors rather than pale pastels (Jordon, 1979). For best results, these bright colors should be incorporated with lighter tones to provide a functional, yet warm, environment.

Sicurella (1977) writes "even the complete absence of glare and the most appropriate lighting, though unquestionably necessary, may do little to help visually impaired persons to see an object if there is insufficient color contrast." In a congregate setting's activity room, two pieces of contact paper can be attached to different surfaces, one dark and one light; older adults with impaired vision can use the dark surface to contrast with a light project and a light surface to contrast with a dark project. For example, when older adults assemble jigsaw puzzles care should be given to contrast table surface with the puzzle pieces.

To facilitate dining, light-colored dinnerware and a dark tablecloth can be used when serving dark foods, and dark dinnerware and a light colored tablecloth when serving light colored foods. Patterned tablecloths, which tend to confuse the eye, should be avoided (Sicurella, 1977). For maximum benefits, dishes, placemats, and tablecloth should all contrast with each other.

Color contrast is helpful in many activities of daily living (Bowersox, 1978), as evidenced by the desirability of having clothing items clearly contrast with each other. Further functioning can be made easier by creating a contrast between the toothbrush and the sink, the slippers and the floor, shirt and sweater, the cookies and the plate, the handrail and the wall.

For the aged person who has difficulty in distinguishing boundaries, the use of color and/or texture differences can clarify such boundaries. For example, the color of the wall and floor should contrast and carpet should not be run up the wall.

Different perceptual tasks are involved in the opacity, transparency, and reflectivity of objects. Contrasts are crucial to being able to see an object well. It has been demonstrated that contrast (the comparison of an object's reflectance with its background reflectance) so greatly affects visual acuity and visual performance (speed and accuracy) that, in many circumstances, contrast in visual task is more important than level of illumination. Other research has demonstrated that performance under low illumination with certain color-rendering qualities can be as good as performance under high illumination with poor color rendition (Lang et al., 1974). Colors appear different according to the surface texture and the amount of light (Hiatt, 1987). When beige, pastel yellow, and pale green are used without the addition of texture on/in walls, bedspreads, or drapery, there may be little differentiation.

Creating a beneficial psychological response through the use of color is a controversial topic. Studies have reported that certain responses can elicit certain behaviors. Reaction to color is based on our cultural background, lighting, texture, and other less obvious interactions. "We cannot arbitrarily say that a color will produce a given effect in behavior of all patients until research accounts for the interactive effect of all these variables" (Hiatt, 1984, pg. 18).

Color scheme can make use of both cool and warm color ranges. One is not limited to red, orange, yellow, or rose. Blue and green tones can be just as effective. When designing living situations for the elderly, the goal in color design is not only to make an area more aesthetically pleasing, but also to help contrast different areas or to be able to distinguish objects from their backgrounds.

Color Coding

The boldness of color coding should be striking enough to convey differences among other elements in the immediate surroundings. Because of the yellowed lens in the older eye, blues may be perceived by the elderly as green. If color is being used to enhance orientation in the long-term care setting, care should be taken to avoid painting adjacent corridors the same shade of blue or green.

One must also be aware of pattern, when dealing with color coding. Many large graphics are beyond the older persons' visual field when they move close enough to discern the detail (Hiatt, 1979). Graphics may enforce an institutional feeling. Also items that surround a person need to have meaning for that individual. Using large graphic patterns for orientation is difficult because they have no cultural meaning for the older person. The importance of the meaning of objects has been discussed in the section on environmental attributes. Different styles of furniture, combined with a particular picture or wall hanging, give a significant cue of a certain floor or area and may be not only more aesthetically acceptable but are items that have more meaning for the individual. In a nursing home, familiar cultural cues, such as a barber pole by a barber shop, are helpful.

In the institutional setting, color coding can provide clear cues for orientation and safety, as well as serving to break the monotony of long halls and large spaces. Color coding has been experimented with in many different ways. Through the use of visual cuing, an area can be made safer and more understandable. In a study done by Liebowitz and Lawton (1979) at the Weiss Institute in Philadelphia, beneficial use of color contrast in the design was reported. Bright colors occurred frequently as accents in door jambs, nursing stations, graphics and room decor. Cooper (1986) implemented a study regarding the effect of color cuing on the functioning level of the institutionalized elderly. She demonstrated the favorable effect of enriching the environment with specific placement of color and light.

Reducing unnecessary information in the corridor of a nursing home can be facilitated through the use of color. Doorways that have no function for the residents, e.g., storage, linen rooms, and locker rooms may be painted the background color of the walls.

Color cuing for directional purpose may not be as effective as object cues. The shape of an object, unusual architecture, a large plant, a window with a view, as well as smells, air currents, and tactile cues all give the older person spatial input. Color is simply one of many ways in which we place, and it should be used in conjunction with texture, shapes, and lighting (Cristarella, 1977; Hiatt, 1979).

Depth Perception

Depth perception depends on brightness and contrast, so any age-related process that affects the amount of light reaching the retina also affects depth perception (Birren, 1977). In fact, one study by Hiatt (1979) indicated that impairment in distance vision was more common than the problem of acuity.

Visual perception studies in the elderly, utilizing various illusion images, indicate that older people tend to retain their original perception and are either resistant or unable to reorganize that perception. Aged subjects also tend to show less "flexibility" in their judgements and poorer performance in gaining information from complex visual designs (Corso, 1971).

Many of these studies used tests emphasizing figure-ground perceptions. These illusions are perceptual fluctuations in which an object or figure may suddenly be perceived as background and the background as a figure. The ability to recognize a simple visual figure when it is embedded in a complex figure background is also difficult (Comalli, 1967). Studies in contrast sensitivity suggest that it may be more difficult for an older individual to discern an object on a surface with an intense pattern background (Owen, 1985).

Compensating for figure-ground problems with the elderly has specific implications when selecting floor covering. As we age, we rely on color in floor surfaces or steps or obstacles. Sometimes these detailed outlines of objects cannot be seen because of loss of depth perception. When pattern is present, as on a floor surface, it may appear to be one object or several objects (Carroll, 1978). The avoidance of patterns on floor surfaces (including stripes, checks, and designs), particularly in hallways, living rooms, or dining rooms, is strongly recommended (Hiatt, 1980).

Owen (1985) reported that the interaction between contrast sensitivity and self motion that is involved in an individual's ability to discriminate objects in a cluttered environment has as yet not been investigated. Therefore the contribution that floor pattern has on the incidence of falls can only be postulated. Research into this area could establish guidelines for carpet manufacturers.

Patterned floors pose additional difficulties for older people who are cognitively impaired. They may perceive patterns as objects but not be able to ask questions or otherwise determine what features are present in an environment. This author and other researchers (Comalli, 1965, 1967) have observed older persons "stepping over" or reaching for support when figure-ground surfaces with excessive contrast sensitivity are present.

Depth perception problems are also manifested through difficulty in distinguishing boundaries (corners where walls meet, the junction of the floor and wall, the level of floors at elevator stops or the edge of a door and the wall in which it is located). In these situations, contrasting colors can help to alleviate depth perception problems.

Other Considerations

In the environment of the person with senile dementia, what is not included visually is also an important consideration. To redirect the confused older adult, doorways have been camouflaged with barriers or room dividers. These screens prevent the confused person from perceiving the exits. Since those who are confused will often follow others, care should be taken by anyone living or working with the older adult as to how they enter and leave the unit. In a study to determine the most effective visual barriers to prevent ambulatory Alzheimer's patients from exiting through an emergency door, the study demonstrated that concealing the doorknob behind a cloth panel was the most successful (Namazi et al., 1989).

Another sign of vision difficulties in the elderly involves the cornea. As a person ages, an opaque ring often forms just inside the cornea. The ring results in reduced peripheral vision because only diffuse light can pass through the opacity (Colavita, 1978). In order to be seen by someone who experiences decreased peripheral vision and low vision, one must enter that person's visual field. This may require being within 18 to 20 inches of the person. The importance of coming very close to the visually impaired older person cannot be over-emphasized.

Even eyeglasses may be a problem. Many visually impaired individuals are unable to clean their own glasses. The build-up of sticky fingerprints can result in visual alterations that render glasses virtually useless, so daily cleaning should be provided by caregivers. Bows need tightening every three to six months. Moreover, bifocals are designed to offer comfortable reading sight, but they may hinder walking because they blur the feet and ground (Wolanin, 1981).

HEARING ADAPTATION

Hearing loss may have an even greater psychological influence on a person than loss of vision. Those who suffer from hearing loss often report feeling unrelated to the world around them. In many cases, depression has been found to overwhelm both the suddenly deafened or those in whom deafness develops gradually (Wolanin, 1981). Indeed, the inability to distinguish words clearly can lead to rejection and withdrawal—either self-inflicted or imposed by others.

Three kinds of hearing loss result in hearing impairment: conductive, sensorineural, and central. These types of loss can occur alone or in combination. In conductive hearing loss, the intensity is not great enough for the sound to reach the inner ear. Increasing the intensity (louder speech or mechanical amplification with a hearing aid) may restore the ability to hear. A central hearing impairment arises when the auditory nerve centers within the brain are affected. These hearing changes may occur at any age. In the elderly, the most common source of auditory problems is a sensorineural loss known as presbycusis.

Presbycusis

Presbycusis is caused by damage to the nerve endings and auditory hair cells in the inner ear. Compounding the problem of hearing perception, for individuals over 75 years of age, is the addition of a reduction in certain auditory nerve cells (Corso, 1971).

These combined losses result in difficulty in hearing high frequency sounds such as a high pitched voice or a shrill whistle. High frequency problems also arise from the inability to discern certain consonants (p, s, th, k, ha, s, sh, and ch) because consonants carry less acoustic power than vowels (Corso, 1971). Because of these two factors, the older individual is unable to discriminate between phonetically similar words making it difficult to follow normal conversation.

Meier (1978, pg. 6F) reported that older persons may hear words as if they sat on top of each other. "Instead of hearing, 'How are you feeling today?' the older person may hear, 'Howareyoufeelingtoday?'" Waiting a second or two for the blurred message to be processed and repeating the information slowly and distinctly will make it easier for the older person to understand what has been said. Rewording sentences also may be helpful when consonants are misunderstood.

The volume maintained for radio, television, and music in any older adult's living situation should be assessed carefully. If volume and treble is increased in relation to the bass, the listener is exposed to overload in the lower tones. Individual adjustment of the treble and bass may compensate for loss of high frequency. Generally, persons with presbycusis are aided if the bass is turned up and the treble is turned down (Hiatt, 1979). This may require routing sound through a more sophisticated stereo system. Because of distortions, music in a high key serves to frustrate and distract rather than relax the person with presbycusis (Hatton, 1977). Music groups that perform in any type of congregate settings should ideally not include flutes and high soprano tones. Speakers and entertainers should be encouraged to use a microphone since this not only amplifies sound but also cuts out some of the high frequencies, making it easier for the person with presbycusis to hear. Sound amplification should be available on all telephones used by the hearing impaired.

Hearing Aids

Attitudes toward hearing aids have changed dramatically in the last few years. One reason for this change is the hearing aid's improved appearance. However, the technology that allows smaller and smaller hearing aids has mixed blessings for the older person. Unfortunately, the operation of smaller hearing aids requires a fine hand and finger dexterity and that is often beyond the physical capacities of older persons.

The recent advances in hearing aid design have been quite remarkable and many persons who previously were not candidates for an aid can now be helped. A hearing aid should not be purchased without an audiological examination. Federal law requires a trial period to determine if the person will benefit from the device.

Hearing aids that compensate for the lost ability to perceive high frequency sounds have been difficult to design. Technologies have been developed that will dampen certain frequencies and thus allow amplifications of only predetermined ranges. Although technically these new designs have tremendous potential the setting of the device may be difficult for the older person. The future development of these devices is quite positive.

Because of the complex nature of presbycusis, some older persons with this disorder receive only partial benefits from using a hearing aid. An aid may only make the distortion louder. Older adults should be made aware that an aid is just a mechanical device and that it has certain limitations.

Some older adults may not use hearing aids because of old batteries, improper fit, and lack of effectiveness. They may need assistance to insert the aid correctly, clean the earmold, or change the batteries.

Assistive listening devices may be used where hearing aids are not effective. These devices are not designed for continuous wear. They consist of microphone and earphones. To use such a device, the older person places the earphones over the ears with the microphone placed close to the desired source of sound (e.g., speech and music). The sound then reaches the ear directly and background noise is reduced. Information concerning the availability of these devices may be obtained from an audiologist, local hearing association, or many stores that carry optical equipment.

Background Noise and Communication

Many elderly people with impaired hearing are reluctant to eat in restaurants or attend large social gatherings because they cannot enjoy the conversation of people around them and, therefore, feel isolated. In rooms where conversational interaction is desired, background sound needs to be reduced. The sound from dishes, fans, television, traffic, music, greatly interferes with the older person hearing pertinent speech. In the institutional setting, intercoms should be used as little a possible because this type of sound produces additional background interference. In dining rooms, persons with an identified hearing loss should not be placed near the kitchen or other noisy areas. In any group, an older person should not be placed on the periphery.

Moving into the field of vision and getting the person's attention before starting to speak are essential elements in communicating with the hearing-impaired person. To facilitate lip reading, one should look directly at the person and speak slowly and distinctly. Shouting is not only unnecessary but causes mouth distortions which make lip reading more difficult.

Older people may also have difficulty locating and identifying the source of sound. The inability to distinguish warning sounds creates tremendous insecurity. This problem, coupled with presbycusis, makes it imperative that fire and smoke alarms, which usually have a high frequency sound, should also have a visual cue, such as a flashing light. Furthermore, inability to determine the source of a sound can create auditory illusions (Wolanin, 1981).

All older adults should have ultimate control over their televisions and/or radio. When used intermittently and purposefully, such media can increase the total amount of stimulation. Radios and television are ideally used to provide a focus for socialization (Wolanin & Phillips, 1981). However, if television is in use continually its sound becomes simply one more channel of background noise. In the institutional setting, this could be accomplished by establishing a schedule of television preferences and usage, with input provided by the residents. It is also important that the administrator and staff become sensitive to the problems created by overload of auditory sensory input. Snyder (1978), demonstrated that wandering and confusion increased in nursing homes during shift changes and other periods of high noise level.

In designing a nursing home's "Alzheimer's Unit," agitation can be addressed by decreasing the background noise. One unit selected for study had a minimum of extra traffic. As part of its design, television sets, the intercom or public address system, and ringing phones were eliminated. No medications were passed at mealtime and residents ate in small groups, reducing noises that were related to the traditional dining room (Hall, 1986). One of the greatest differences between home and the long-term care facility is the accoustical environment. "Poorly managed and designed accoustical settings can be as great a barrier to older people as steps are to a wheelchair user" (Hiatt, 1985, pg. 16).

Residences can be designed, however, to alleviate acoustical distractions. Furnishings and materials that absorb sound, reduce echoes, and muffle irrelevant noise can be introduced. The use of acoustical ceiling tile is usually the most economical and effective way to lower sound levels but carpeting, draperies, and other upholstery fabrics also reduce noise levels. Decorative baffles and wall hangings reduce background noise and add aesthetic visual appeal (Bowersox, 1979).

Insulating sheetrock should be installed around noisy areas, such as kitchens, living rooms, or maintenance and mechanical rooms. Tight window weather seals reduce exterior sound noise. On the exterior, earth berms, trees and large plant material will assist in diverting and absorbing traffic sounds. Such acoustic landscaping is of particular value in an urban setting (Bowersox, 1979).

Within the long-term care facility, sounds can be cues to certain locations. Screening out helpful sounds, such as those from the activity room, lounge, or beauty shop, may not be necessary or desireable. Each area must be examined in light of the residents diagnosis for that particular space (Koncelik, 1976).

UTILIZING TASTE AND SMELL

Taste

The sense of taste consists of four components-sweet, salty, bitter, and sour—all of which are chemically induced. Schiffman (1975) suggests a decline in sensitivity with age for each of these gustatory qualities, although certain studies indicate an increased response to bitterness. Furthermore, some research suggests more of a decline in salty sensitivity in males (Corso, 1971). Medications, dentures and certain diseases also have an impact on the sense of taste. However, it appears that changes in the gustatory system do not seriously affect the sense of taste until relatively late in life.

Those who provide food service to the elderly need to be reminded of the sensory changes occurring in the aged because of the importance of the dining experience. Many caregivers report an increase in the use of condiments, particularly sugar and salt. However, these additions create problems because so many residents have either a salt or sugar-restricted diet. Therefore, the dietitian needs to find safe substitutes, such as a variety of herbs and spices, in order to provide greater taste satisfaction for the older person.

While the sense of taste is not an intricate part of environment cuing, it can be utilized for specific gustatory stimulation, such as tasting parties, e.g., wine, cheese, and ice cream. When an ethnic dinner is served, food is combined with music, costumes, dances and visual effects.

Smell

The olfactory sense provides protection and pleasure. It can generate associations of ideas and past experiences. Aromas of fresh-mown hay and rain-soaked sod conjure up more than smells. Helen Keller utilized her keen sense of smell to identify people. Moreover, two-thirds of the response to taste lies in the sense of smell (Ernst, 1976). The aroma of food changes mere acceptance into appreciation of flavor.

The literature on olfactory sensitivity is contradictory, but sensation appears to decrease with age (Busse, 1978). Besides a reduction in the pleasure of pleasant smells, the older person may have a reduced sensitivity to body and household odors that may be offensive to others. A loss in olfaction also seems to hinder the ability to smell smoke or gas fumes. In an English study conducted by Chalke (1957), 892 deaths by domestic gas poisoning were examined. Results showed that over 75% of those who died were over 60 years of age.

The early analysis of the National Geographic Smell Survey conducted in 1986 showed a noticeable decline in the ability to detect scents at age 70 and a significant decline at age 80. One potential problem area that was revealed by this survey, involves the addition of mercaptains (foul smelling additives), to natural gas that warn of leaks. "Asked to comment on the odor's unpleasantness, older respondents showed surprising lack of strong negative reaction, possibly indicating unsuitability of the smell as a warning of danger" (Gilbert & Wysocki, 1987, pg. 522).

Long-term care organizations must be alert to the impact of smells in a facility. Smells can linger in draperies and other fabrics long after the immediate cause of the odor has been eliminated.

Opportunities also exist to increase good smells. Popcorn and coffee produce familiar odors. The smell of baking, flowers and plants, and fresh air need to be incorporated into any and all design projects. Plants that are colorful and fragrant should be placed, both inside and outside the living environment. In settings which house confused residents, plants must be of a non-poisonous variety (Bowersox, 1979).

TACTILE/TOUCH CONCERNS

Sensory input through the skin is subdivided into the touch and the tactile systems. An individual's system utilizes touch for awareness and protective responses and tactile input to interact with the environment. These tactile receptors allow us to perceive multiple characteristics of an object (Huss, 1977). For example, a wet rock could be cold, hard, and smooth (Walker, 1972). According to researchers, the major touch/tactile changes occurring with aging, which have implications for environmental design, are in the areas of tactile discrimination (Montagu, 1978).

Tactile Input

The response to a decrease in discriminatory input may take a number of forms. Such responses might include: avoiding participation in activities involving tactile discrimination, holding an object with an unusually strong grasp, having items slip from the hand or increasing feeling of items with texture. These changes, as in all sensory systems, may occur gradually or not at all (Ernst, 1976).

The importance of tactile input may at first appear contradictory. When other senses are impaired, particularly vision and hearing, the older person relies more on the tactile sense. However, with aging there are decreases in this response to tactile input. Thus, to assist the older person, the degree and variety of texture needs to be increased (Birren, 1977). This can be very beneficial in the corridor of the long-term care facility.

However, care should be taken when introducing texture into smaller areas. Too much variation of texture in a small lounge or resident room should be avoided. Textures as well as other color schemes should be carefully combined so as not to overload the individual. One dominant texture in an area is more effective than many combining varied textures (Koncelik, 1976). Coarse wall hangings made from burlap, carpet, heavy yarns, or rope will add interesting texture. Carpeting, velour, textured upholstery, and wood, not only cut down on glare, but add warmth and tactile input. Vinyl wall covering is easy to maintain and increases the tactile "readability" with definite texture. Cost can be decreased and texture increased by combining smooth painted surfaces with vinyl wall covering (Bowersox, 1979). Varied floor coverings likewise increase the degree of texture in an area. Outdoors, a distinctive surface treatment can be used to guide the older person to a particular seating area. Living spaces designed for the older adult should be assessed carefully for positive effects of varied textures in the architectural design. Large pillars, alcoves in a corridor area, and landmarks can help orient persons regarding location. The addition of items such as plants, grandfather clocks, umbrella racks, and resident mailboxes add richness and tactile variety to the environment.

Variations on the surface of handrails, such as knurling or

grooves, give cues to turns or the approaching end of a wall. Furthermore, fire and exterior doorknobs are required to have some type of textural surface for safety purposes.

In institutional settings, to allow for a variety of textures against the skin, residents should be encouraged to wear street clothes rather than institutional garments. Surrounding a person with a variety of fabrics, such as soft blankets and textured towels can eliminate total tactile deprivation.

Large raised (or recessed) letters and numbers are more effective than braille identification for the elderly person with severe sight impairment (Bowersox, 1978). Most visually impaired elderly have never learned braille, and when there is tactile loss the texture of braille may not be varied enough to serve as identification.

When temperature sensitivity occurs in older persons, most people report a greater susceptibility to cold than to heat (Birren, 1977). Older persons often require lap robes and sweaters in temperature settings that appear quite warm to the younger person (Carroll, 1978). Outdoor environments should be protected from breezes with fences or baffles.

Touch

Many researchers note the elderly person's need to be touched. Touch enhances the feeling of well-being, but as people age, they have fewer significant others with whom touching is acceptable behavior. "One has only to observe the responses of older people to a caress, an embrace, a hand-pat or a clasp, to appreciate how vitally necessary such experiences are for their well-being" (Montagu, 1978, pg. 321). Animals and children add considerably to touch input in the environment.

Caregivers may need to learn the importance of using a caring touch with the elderly, as well as learning to give and receive touch comfortably (Huss, 1977). Occasionally an aversion to being touched may be present because of certain physiological, cultural, and social factors. Those who care for older adults must be aware that this can occur, and should use touch at the level that is comfortable for the older person (Wolanin, 1981).

For the seriously ill or confused, touch is a valuable communication tool. To investigate the effects of touch with seriously ill patients, one study compared a group of subjects who were touched while talking with the study's investigator to a control group who were not touched. The findings demonstrated that use of touch showed seriously ill patients that the nurse cared about them (McCorkle, 1974). In fact, as a person's length of stay in the nursing home increases and he/she establishes closer ties to the nursing staff, touch deprivation may actually become less severe. Emotion, perception, motivation, drive, wakefulness and sleep are all associated with neurological and brain activity as well as outside stimuli (Noback, 1975).

One other important aspect of touch in the nursing home is the attachment to meaningful objects. Personal items take on special importance to the long-term care resident. Huss (1977) relates a study where the elderly clung to possessions they could handle or possessions that evoked memories. Multiple studies on reminiscence and life review lend credence to this observation. In the section on environmental attributes there is an indepth discussion of the meaning the older person may attach to objects.

KINESTHETIC INPUT

Kinesthesia, the position and balance sense, has two groups of sensors. The proprioceptive sense is located in the joints and deep tissue of the limbs and indicates the position of body parts in space. The major age-related problems in proprioception result in: (1) decreased ability to judge an object's weight, (2) decreased awareness of the position of body parts which is coupled with other musculoskeletal changes and (3) decreased coordination and speed of contraction (Birren, 1977). This decreased feedback in proprioception results in deficits in motor coordination because perception of body movement is critical to performing skilled activities.

The vestibular portion of the inner ear gives input concerning an individual's head position. The older person with changes in the vestibular system has a decrease in the ability to determine when and in what direction the head is moving. This leads to an increase in the possibility of falling (Hasselkus, 1974). Environmental adaptation can compensate for certain losses in these senses.

Proprioception

Proprioceptive changes cause the elderly to move more slowly. The step of older persons is shorter, higher, and wider-based, with more time spent in support before the next move is made; thus, the older person should never be rushed when walking (Murray et al., 1969; Finely et al., 1969). They should, however, be involved in activities that provide moderate amounts of physical activity. Proprioceptive response is essential to perform activities of daily living. Additional input can be encouraged by providing walking, dancing, and exercise groups (Richman, 1969).

Hiatt (1979) has indicated that many falls can be traced to the older person's sudden weight shift in relation to a mirror-like waxed floor. Such falls may be exaggerated by osteoporosis, cardiovascular disorders, muscular weakness, and, of primary concern in this section, dizziness and decreased input from the muscle and joint receptors (Birren, 1977).

The cause of all falls needs to be determined, and the possibility of environmental interventions needs to be evaluated. Although floor surfaces were mentioned in a previous section, further comments are necessary.

Floor Covering

Of the various types of floor covering on the market, vinyl composition tile (VCT), sheet vinyl, and carpet are the most popular. VCT accommodates wheelchair traffic, is relatively inexpensive to install and has adequate color choices. However, it also requires extensive maintenance, is noisy, produces glare and has an institutional appearance. Sheet vinyl on the other hand accommodates wheelchair traffic, is more expensive to install, has good color choices, and requires medium-high maintenance.

Carpet has approximately the same installation price as sheet vinyl but produces more drag on the wheels, which may cause difficulties for some wheelchair users. Carpet also requires that spills be cleaned immediately. Overall, though, a feeling of warmth and comfort is projected by carpet; it is quiet, traps air-born bacteria dust; and has a wide color and texture range. Older adults also appear to feel more secure on carpet. Gait speed and step length have been demonstrated to be significantly greater on carpet than on a vinyl surface (Willmott, 1986). Although installation costs for VCT are the least expensive, user-cost comparison shows carpet, over the lifetime of the product, to be less expensive (Reznikoff, 1979). Maintenance of carpet and vinyl flooring are entirely different, but either one can be used in most areas accommodating older individuals. Carpet squares have been successfully used in some situations, particularly in high traffic areas where they can be easily replaced at minimal expense.

The older adult's floor surface should also be free of unnecessary obstacles. Throw rugs, door thresholds and trailing telephone and extension cords should be eliminated.

Ambulation Aids

Handrails should be placed on both sides of the hall since ambulatory elderly may have use of only one side, e.g., after a stroke or because of neurological involvement or amputation. Observations of ambulation in nursing homes have shown that only a minority of ambulatory residents actually use the hand rail for assistance while walking. In these settings, handrails are used primarily by the person in a wheelchair who pulls him/herself down the hall using the handrail as an ambulatory assist. Koncelik (1976) has suggested that ideally there should be two handrails on the same wall, one placed at 32 inches and the other at approximately 26 inches, to allow for use by both the ambulatory and nonambulatory person. The shape of the handrail itself is also a consideration. Handrails should be selected which provide the older hand with comfortable grasp and maximum safety. The best handrail design is cylindrical in shape and 1 1/4 to 1 1/2 inches in diameter.

Some type of support should also be available through open areas, as in dining rooms, living rooms, and day rooms. Tables should be sturdy because most older people will use them either for support when rising from a chair or for balance when walking.

If older adults are using stairs, a four-inch height is preferable to the usual eight inches. Women, in particular, tend to "let down" from one step to the next with a jarring motion, so a shallower step lessens the likelihood of injury (Hasselkus, 1974).

Balance

Muscle tone and postural adjustment also are dependent upon the vestibular system. Injury to the inner ear and the auditory nerve has consequences other than total deafness. Flabbiness of the neck, limb, and trunk muscles along with disturbed action of the eye muscles are likely to occur (Gelard, 1953). Decreased strength in the postural muscles of the trunk may lead to a reduction of balance and equilibrium reactions. Whereas, the younger person merely tilts forward to maintain balance, the older person has a decreased ability to determine when the body is tilting. Thus, adjustments in posture are required and this often leads to falls.

Postural changes include a forward shift in the center of gravity resulting in greater body weight on the toes. Because of postural changes, the older adult may find it easier and safer to negotiate stairs rather than ramps (Hiatt, 1979). Although a ramp is required for the wheelchair user, certain hazards exist for ramp usage in the long-term care facility. For the older ambulatory adult, the combined effects of that person's lowered gaze, forward tilt due to osteoporosis, and incline of the ramp may all contribute to a dangerous alteration in balance when the person is walking down the ramp.

The older wheelchair user may also have some difficulty with ramps. Because of reduced upper extremity strength in the elderly, ramps may be too steep for the older person to negotiate. Any ramp for the older adult should have a pitch of 1:20 rather than the accessibility standard of 1:12.

Those who care for impaired older adults should use caution when moving the wheelchair-bound person. The change in the ability to process vestibular information may make the world appear to be moving much faster than it is and this can create fear for the impaired individual.

Although disturbances in the vestibular system may cause dizziness, other problems may also contribute to such a reaction. For example, a person may have arteriosclerotic changes of the blood vessels of the neck and/or deterioration of neck vertebrae resulting in reduced arterial flow. Both processes may create problems in circulation to the brain. Dizziness or even unconsciousness may occur when the person turns his neck or looks upward. Therefore older persons should be cautioned not to make quick head motions either from side to side or upward and not to sit or stand with their head tipped back for a prolonged period of time. These conditions give further credence to placing signs and directional information at their proper heights as well as the necessity for not locating the television set high on the wall. The seated older person needs the set placed near eye-level.

Changes in posture due to osteoporosis are another reason for lower sign placement. Even to compensate for vision and hearing deficits, residents should not be seated at a movie, concert, or religious service, in a position requiring the head to be tipped back for a prolonged time. The height of clothing rods and shelves in closets, and the location of a television set should take into consideration the effect on head position. Because of the difficulty in turning the head from side to side, these limitations also reduce social interaction when people are seated next to each other on benches or sofas. Socialization increases when persons are seated at right-angles to each other.

Antibiotics that cause hearing loss also affect the vestibular portion of the inner ear and may cause dizziness. Prolonged use of these drugs should be monitored.

Tactile, kinesthetic, and vestibular stimulation have been relatively unexplored with regard to the elderly. Even recognition of the importance of touch to normal development and adequate functioning at earlier stages is fairly recent. Research by Kramer and Piermont (1976) has documented that preterm infants rocked mechanically on waterbeds and given auditory stimulation gained significantly more weight than nonstimulated infants. Harlow's experiments with rhesus monkeys deprived of touch and kinesthetic stimulation showed that these monkeys resorted to body rocking in the same way as human children, raised in institutions, who were touched and cared for infrequently (Montagu, 1978).

Rocking behavior is commonly seen in the disoriented elderly. Is this self-induced movement an attempt to increase vestibular stimulation? The need for self-determined vestibular input can be encouraged by including rocking chairs in the person's environment. Outdoor porches are a good investment for resident well-being, particularly if porch swings and rocking chairs are included. If swings are used, the arm of the swing should be part of the support system of the chair and not moveable.

CONCLUSION

In our twentieth century society, alert, active "senior citizens" have become commonplace. However, the homes of these independent seniors may have potential hazards that need to be assessed to determine interventions which will maximize their functioning. Residents as well as managers of senior housing are extremely reluctant to include interventions, such as handrails in corridors or grab bars in bathrooms, that are construed to convey less than total independence. These individuals need information regarding the benefits of including unobtrusive and yet specific adaptations that will promote independence.

"The nursing home environment must project a 'can do' image. The atmosphere must promote independence rather than dependence and at all times should accommodate the deficits of normal aging" (Erickson, 1989, pg. 18). In the long-term care facility the input of the staff is essential if these design interventions are to have optimal effect. In a study done by Hanley (1981) the orientation of residents was improved through the active involvement of the caregivers. Sights, sounds, smells, and textures in the environment should be used to relate to the residents.

Regardless of the setting, sensory impairment can be compensated for, to some degree, if the environment is designed and modified to allow individuals to operate at their maximum potential. With greater knowledge, planning and conscious effort, environments that stimulate, work for, and respond to the sensory needs of the older person can be a reality.

Designing for the Older Person by Addressing Environmental Attributes

INTRODUCTION

The importance of the environment is often overlooked, perhaps because of the obvious nature of the interplay between behavior and environment. An individual's behavior in a space is directly related to the design of that space, therefore environment can not be studied separately from behavior (Ittelson et al., 1970). Because activity and environment cannot be separated, the environment for the elderly must be designed in such a way that optimum functioning can take place.

As a way to study this interaction between the older person and their environment, environmental press and competence have been examined by Lawton and Nahemow (1973). They stipulated that adaptive behavior is a joint function of competence and environmental press which creates a person/environment interdependence. Competence is based on physical reserve, endurance, stamina, and strength. Because different environments place different demands, the level of adaptation varies. Environmental press is the demand placed upon us under varying circumstances. The "adaptation level" defines the point at which positive outcomes occur with little awareness of environmental press. This "adaptation level" is a balance between competence and environmental demand.

When environmental demands slightly exceed the adaptation level a stimulating environment is created. If environmental demands surpass the individuals competence to cope, stress occurs. If the environment is not stimulating enough, sensory deprivation can be the result. Design that adapts for the changes that occur with aging is crucial in providing an environment in which the older person can function to the maximum of his or her competence. The environment as a "hidden modality" (Kiernat, 1982) cannot be overlooked. The therapist can utilize the environment as part of a well-conceived treatment plan.

In designing environments for older persons we must be aware that competence is impacted by many psychological and social factors. These less tangible factors deal with environmental characteristics that must be met to truly allow a person to age well in the designed environment. These characteristics have been described as environmental attributes (Windley & Scheidt, 1980), which ascribe both a social and physical component to a particular item or place. In this section, a variety of these attributes will be discussed, as well as how we are impacted by them and ways that they can be incorporated into the living settings of the older person.

In younger years, for the person who can live where he or she chooses, most of these sought after qualities are satisfied. For the older person who may not be able to live in the place he or she prefers, attention to providing these environmental attributes has potential to maximize functioning and provide more flexibility.

Resident satisfaction was examined in a study by Weidemann et al. (1982). The two most important predictors of resident satisfaction were the attractiveness of the facility and their perceptions of safety and security. The second most important predictor of resident satisfaction contained items about the amount of comfort, space and economic value of the apartment.

Although these environmental characteristics are important to each one of us regardless of the place where we live, for a variety of reasons some aspects have more impact than others. Concern about forced entry will cause greater anxiety for the individual in a single family dwelling in a high crime area than for the person living in a nursing home in a low crime area. Privacy is more of an issue for the person who shares a room in a long-term care facility than it is for the individual living in their own unit in a senior residence. Ways to personalize spaces in a resident room in a nursing home are more limited than personalization of an apartment or unit in senior housing.

This discussion addresses the following attributes: comfort, legibility, privacy, accessibility, adaptability, meaning, control, density, security and dignity, aesthetics and sensory stimulation. Many of these attributes are closely related and a product or space may need to address more than one environmental attribute. For instance, a comfort factor is assessed by asking: "Does the chair provide comfort for older persons over an extended period of time?" "Does the position of the arms of the chair allow for ease in getting in and out?" focuses on accessibility.

The inclusion of these attributes into housing for the older person provides a base for autonomy by allowing the person more control of his/her environment. It must be emphasized, however, that in the traditional nursing home environment, autonomy is highly dependent upon the staff and their interactions with the resident. The environment can be designed to promote independence and control but the staff must respect this need and attempt to care for the needs of the resident with these autonomous concerns in mind. In a study of residents in an old-age home (Saup, 1987), it was determined that stress-reducing coping behavior would be facilitated by reducing uncontrollable environmental features, such as standardized rooms and not possessing a house-key, by means of environmental planning.

SENSORY STIMULATION

Controversy often exists concerning the amount of sensory stimulation that should be provided for the older person. Although there is a reduction in sensory information received by an older individual (Lawton & Nahemow, 1973) and information may often be processed more slowly (Eisdorfer, 1968), there is still a great deal of variability amongst individuals and what is too much for one person may not be enough for another.

Part of the complexity of designing supportive environments for the elderly is the necessity of having to make arbitrary decisions about certain design elements. The optimal level of stimulation for one person may be either too much or too little for another. Individual differences in these optimal levels have existed during the person's entire life. By nature some persons are sensation seekers and others sensation reducers (Wolanin, 1981).

Impacting upon these normal sensation needs are the age-related sensory changes. The amount of light may need to be increased for one individual but for another direct light, particularly when it produces glare, needs to be reduced. When possible, several solutions must be worked into a design plan. In the pioneering work done by Pastalan, Mautz and Merrill (1970), researchers participating in that study experienced cautiousness, disorientation and decreased speed of activity when there was a reduction and distortion of sensory information.

COMFORT

In the designed environment comfort is a subjective quality which furnishes physical ease in doing a task or being in a particular place. The most evident of all of the environmental attributes, to the individual, is the level of comfort. Many of these comfort features are based upon meeting age-related sensory and physical needs. The following are examples of concerns that would be addressed:

- Is the sound level controlled adequately?
- Is the lighting adequate for the individual to be able to read?
- Does the lighting minimize eye strain?
- Is the temperature at a comfortable level?
- Does the furniture "fit" the individual?

Independence can be augmented by designing for the comfort of the older person. Raschko (1982) reminds us that it is better to think of ranges when designing for the elderly than averages. Environmental design should vary from considerations for the small female to the large male both ambulatory and wheelchair user. The application of these concerns will depend on the product and the location. The range these individuals can reach is referred to as the "comfort zone." This area should be the determining factor in the placement of all features, i.e., clothes rods, bottom of kitchen cabinets, electrical outlets and switches, and top of kitchen base cabinets.

As the activity level of the older person decreases, the amount of time spent in a chair increases. Inquiry must be made into the comfort of a particular chair for a specific individual. Often, when designing supportive environments, either senior housing or long-term care facilities, many chairs must be purchased. The challenge of selecting a chair that is comfortable for an individual is compounded by the need to obtain many chairs. An indepth discussion of the design and selection of chairs is included in this publication.

ACCESSIBILITY

Accessibility is first the ease with which a person gets from point A to point B or in and out of certain spaces. Traditionally, therapists concerns with accessibility have focused on the wheelchair user and architectural barriers. Architectural barriers have been defined as "any architectural feature of a facility which make it difficult or impossible for persons with disabilities to use" (AOTA, 1983, pg. 27). For the older person in a wheelchair, all of the traditional accessibility concerns apply.

In the more general context of the designed environment for the elderly, accessibility and the ease with which a person gets from point A to point B or in and out of certain spaces must include not only the person with limited mobility but also the ability and ongoing desire to walk from place to place. Accessibility in this regard includes chair design and the inclusion of chairs along a route to allow for occasional stops. It also includes not only the ability to move about, unhindered, in that environment but also the freedom to perform daily living tasks.

The location of cupboard and closet shelves and drawers to eliminate the need for extensive bending, reaching or strength is a crucial part of making an environment accessible. For drawers, outlets, and shelves Raschko (1983) has described an area of accessibility which extends beyond the defined "comfort area." This area would vary with each individual and, particularly in the designed environment of supportive housing, provide flexibility and adaptability for the items that would lie within this range.

Accessibility also includes the ability to manipulate more stationery objects or products. Within the context of that definition are bathroom/kitchen fixtures. Products such as rocker-type light switches and lever door handles must also be included. The grab bar is a device that can provide accessibility into and out of a tub. However, because most grab bars are stainless steel they have a cold clinical appearance. This look often negatively influences the older persons acceptance of the device. Colored grab bars, which are incorporated with the bathroom decor, may be more readily accepted by the senior.

LEGIBILITY

Windley and Scheidt (1980) remind us that legibility is defined as how clearly information is packaged and portrayed and is affected by how much incoming information the organism is capable of receiving and processing. With reduced sensory input in the elderly, this information may be clouded and even misinterpreted. For the person with dementia and age-related sensory change these misinterpretations can create a variety of illusions. Ways to enhance legibility for the person with dementia must be incorporated into their designed environment.

Legibility enhances predictability and orientation by reducing general ambiguity. Even the alert elderly experience difficulty with ambiguous and intense stimuli or environments that lack unidentifiable components such as streets in a city or corridors in a building (Windley & Scheidt, 1980). In long-term care facilities, legibility is best accomplished through appropriate cues and landmarks. Orientation is facilitated by visually distinctive landmarks and a comprehensible pathway (Christenson & Raschko, 1989).

In a study of persons living in a high rise, those who had difficulty finding their own apartments indicated the problem was caused by uniformity of floor design, lack of personalization of floors and doors and lack of orientation cues (Devlin, 1980). Corridors in senior housing or a long-term care facility often lack these visual cues.

In long term care facilities persons often become lost in the corridor or in finding their way on different floors. When each hallway or floor is designed exactly the same, cues as to a persons location in the space are missing. Designed spaces such as lounges with one-of-type design, a barber shop with a barber pole, a greenhouse, a cabinet to display crafts can aid in orientation. In rural long-term care facilities, if crafts are no longer an integral part of the activities program, this display space can be converted into a display area for familiar farm implements.

If these corridors are lacking in architectural spaces, actual objects such as grandfather clocks, large potted plants, and pianos, can be incorporated. If space is limited, landmarks in the form of pictures must be relied upon to provide legibility. An indepth discussion on the selection of landmarks and signage is included in the section "Redesigning the Long-Term Care Facility."

Predicability for the visually and hearing impaired can be enhanced. For individuals suffering from auditory distortions, sound insulative materials and acoustical materials will reduce reverberations and echos. Incorporating the suggestions which have been discussed in the section on adaptations to compensate for sensory change will increase the predicability for the person with visual impairment.

SECURITY

Security and safety are closely allied. For the independent elderly in their own home, security against forced entry involves concerns for both theft and bodily harm. Surveilance systems and burglar alarms are available at a variety of prices and levels of satisfaction. Creating an environment that minimizes these dangers can not only provide protection and peace of mind, but the reduced anxiety the older person experiences provides encouragement to increase mobility which impacts other attributes such as control, privacy, and accessibility.

Environmental interventions that increase safety can also increase mobility by eliminating hazardous situations such as slippery floors, improperly designed thresholds in doorways, grab bars not secured in the studs or handrails on only one side of stairs. These concerns have been discussed in the section entitled "Enhancing Independence in the Home Setting."

An extendable rail is available which allows those who have difficulty with stairs to use them with increased ease and frequency. This rail is actuated by pulling it from the wall to the extended position, bringing it to within 22 inches of the rail on the other side. A unique locking system provides strength when the rail is either fully extended or folded back against the wall. (See Photograph 1.) The effect is similar to having a walker firmly affixed to the stair-

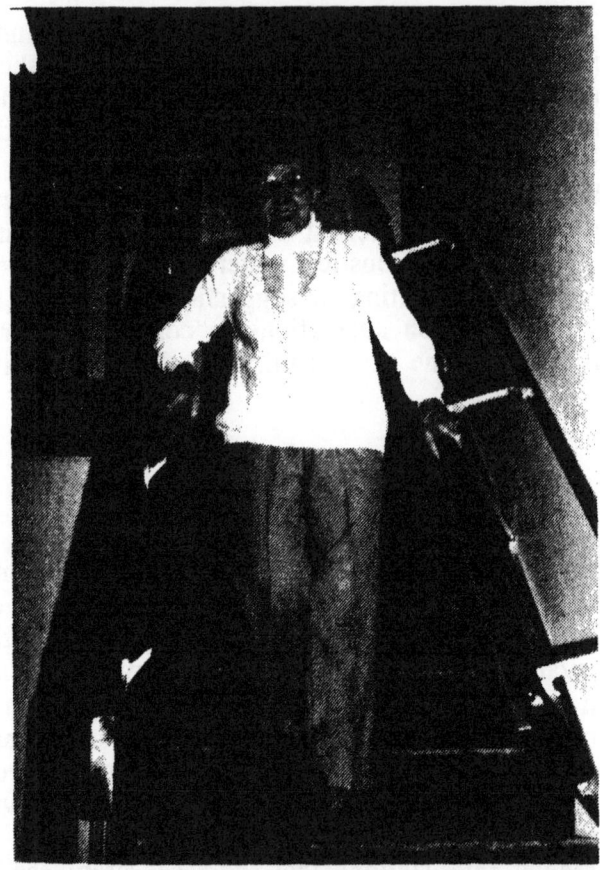

PHOTOGRAPH 1. St. Croix Stair Rail with rail extended

case and allows the the user to use both hands while moving up and
down stairs. This devise is manufactured by St. Croix Rail.

Another somewhat more expensive solution for the stair-user
might be a stair elevator. Some companies do provide rental of
these units. Elevators accommodate almost any type of stairway
and form a self-contained unit.

The emergency response system is a product that can increase a
sense of security. These systems provide 24-hour monitoring and
help people live independently. At the first sign of trouble, a sub-

scriber pushes a button which activates a sequence of calls to provide help from identified informal as well as formal care givers. New models are being developed which can be activated with a cry or loud noise. Traditionally, in senior housing and institutions, wall mounted pull cords have been employed to provide a means for residents to call for help. Unfortunately, accidents often occur out of the range of these cords and although help is available in the building the victim may not be able to notify anyone. In-house emergency systems, similar to those used by the person living independently in his/her home, are now being considered in senior housing.

Aesthetically, well-designed dishes can provide security for the person with weakness or a tremor that limits their ability to eat without spilling. A pattern manufactured by Royal Doulton has a cup with two handles and an edge on the plates that acts as a plate guard. These dishes are not only attractive but if used in a long-term care facility eliminate the frustrations of the misplacement of the plate guard. The use of these products can provide dignity for individuals and, when dining, increase socialization.

More attention must be placed upon the safety features in products used by the older person. Products that offered additional margins of safety would benefit individuals of all ages, but especially older adults at risk. Older people, just as persons in any age group, vary in their physical needs, skill and attention to safety; they do have a higher rate of accidents involving products. To create changes in the design of products will require the involvement of many disciplines plus the crucial input of the older consumer (COMSIS, 1988). In a study done by the Minnesota Gerontological Society (1989) involving a survey of manufacturing and business communities in Minnesota, it was found that communication was lacking between the manufacturers and the elderly users or the therapist that might be prescribing a device.

Safety issues must be paramount when dealing with the person with dementia, particularly in his/her home. Kern (1986) has suggested "Occupational Therapists should establish clear guidelines, develop evaluation criteria and produce practical instruction information regarding environmental safety at home, in the daycare setting and long-term care facilities" (pg. 4).

PRIVACY

Privacy has been defined as an individual's ability to decide what information and under what circumstances a person should communicate. It also is the ability to control unwanted stimuli, primarily visual or auditory. Researchers agree that adequate privacy enhances self-regard and provides opportunities for solitude, self-reflection, and often emotional release (Altman 1974, Pastalan 1970 & Westin, 1970).

Privacy is vital to a sense of autonomy. "Autonomy is a sense of individual and conscious choice in which the person controls his environment, including his ability to have privacy when desired" (Tate, 1980). In a nursing home, the resident's sense of autonomy may be threatened not only by unannounced help from the staff (Nastalan, 1970) but the lack of a place or time when he or she can be alone, particularly for the resident who shares a room. Times of solitude provide us with opportunities for emotional release as well as self-evaluation. In a study by Firestone et al. (1980) it was reported that "ward residents viewed the nursing home as an insecure place affording insufficient privacy and oversufficient accessibility" (pg. 238).

Privacy also allows an older person to make his or her own choices regarding group participation. Often the resident's desire and staff perception of need differ. Opportunities for this type of anonymity must be respected and weighed against an individual's need for socialization. In any discussion of privacy we must be aware that the type or degree of privacy required by an individual may have a strong cultural base (Rullo, 1987). Being cognizant of this fact can help us in our planning of long-term care facilities.

For long-term care facilities the private versus semi-private rooms discussion continues. In a study by Lawton and Bader (1970), persons of varying ages and living situations were interviewed as to their room or projected room preferences. There was no overpowering inclination for private rooms. Those persons already living in the institution were less likely to want a private room than persons living in the community.

Schwartz (1969) reported that in the institutionalized elderly a reduced desire for privacy was correlated with the amount of time in the institution. As the result of an interview with older residents, Pastalan (1986) concluded that as physical capacity decreases, the desire for large rooms also decreased. One man indicated that in the smaller room he was able to get around without a walker. In a larger room he did not think this would be possible. To maximize privacy in the institutional setting, Koncelik (1976) has suggested that all lounges be located between resident rooms and the corridors.

Privacy can be promoted through the design of spaces. In senior housing, visual access into bathrooms and bedrooms from the living room area should be avoided. Although window treatment should provide glare control and allow for a view, it should provide privacy as well. Usually a combination of blinds and drapery is best.

ADAPTABILITY

Ideally elderly environments should be able to be rearranged when the need or desire arises. If the health status of an individual changes can accommodations be made in the current housing that increase the potential for aging in place?

If the individual has difficulty with stairs can either the elevator or extendable rail, (illustrated in Photograph 1 on page 38) be used? If neither of these alternative devices are successful, can the daily living tasks that occurred on the upper floor be rearranged to the first floor? For instance, can a space on the first floor be made into a bedroom? If the bathroom is upstairs and plumbing or cost does not allow for one on the main floor, can a private place for a commode be created on the main floor?

Ideally, when the needs and desires of the older person change, furniture should be designed so it can be rearranged. Studies have shown that some senior housing accommodate large pieces of furniture better than others (Howell, 1980). Moveable storage closets have been designed to provide flexibility and maximize space.

New designs for bath tubs have been developed which can be retrofitted and in place of a standard tub, provide a tub which is entered at chair height. This tub features ease of access and eliminates the necessity of bending. (See Photograph 2.) A unit is also available which is a variation on this tub and has several phases that

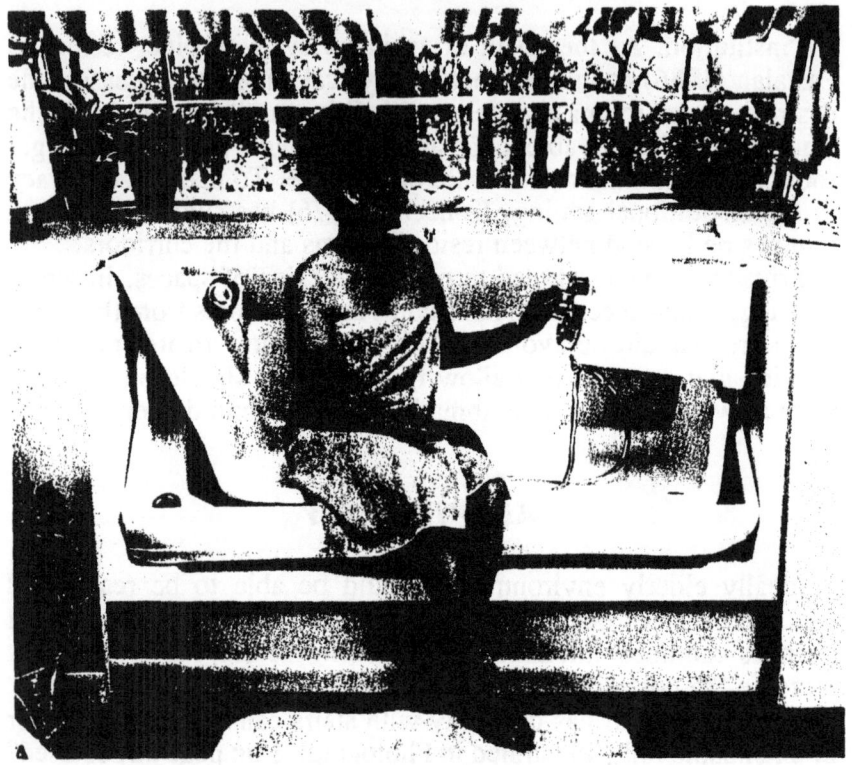

PHOTOGRAPH 2

can adapt to the needs of the older person beginning with a shower and continuing through to the retrofitted tub.

MEANING

Although the meaning of a structure or space is illusive and difficult to measure it has a definite influence upon a persons attitude toward a particular building or space (Windley & Scheidt, 1980). Designers need to be aware that meaning for the older person can be affected by memories associated with intangible design components of places.

The home has particular significance in its relationship to a person's sense of belonging and rootedness (Rullo, 1987). High attachment to a dwelling is most commonly based on number of years of occupancy. O'Bryant (1983) identified subjective factors which correlated with a high level of housing satisfaction. Of these factors three that might be anticipated were, (1) housing cost that was adequate to meet the person's daily needs, (2) the status of being a home owner, and (3) feelings of competence in the familiar environment. The fourth was that the home was seen as a repository of family traditions.

As a person ages, buildings or furniture styles may generate memories, positive or negative, of growing up in a certain kind of house. The response of a person to Victorian, modern or colonial decor may be based on these memories.

In a study of the significance of items, Csikszenthmihalyi and Rochberg-Halton (1981) determined that objects help us develop and maintain our concept of self. They found that older respondents placed greater significance upon photo albums than did middle aged persons. The responses of certain of the older persons to the favorite chair went beyond the comfort factor and dealt with memories about conversations or experiences that occurred around that chair.

Howell (1985) reminds us that organizing personal memories to permit an individual to adjust to a new setting requires considerable thought and effort. When an older person is moving to either senior housing or a nursing home, reducing the number of possessions that will fit in a smaller space is difficult. Assessing personal items in the light of the memories they evoke can help with relocation.

PERSONALIZATION

Personalization allows a person to convey individual ownership of a space and enhances their feelings of security. In designing long-term care facilities, interests of the residents should always be considered. In senior housing, the person's identity may be closely tied to pre-retirement roles. Flexible community and private spaces should be provided for gardening, hobbies, personal computers, musical instruments. In resident units, regardless of the level of care, adequate display and storage space must be provided.

In the nursing home, personalization can be fostered by encouraging the resident to bring a variety of items from their homes to the facility. These may include a chair, bedspread, lamps, radio, television, as well as pictures and other memorabilia. Organizational philosophies vary and is manifested in personalization policies. Some space is provided in almost all nursing homes for the resident to display cards, pictures, and other small items. In a study of residents who had lost possessions they had brought to the nursing home due to a facility fire, it was found that the items which were most difficult to have lost included not only family pictures, photo albums, home furnishings, clothing and jewelry but important papers and holiday decorations (Bell, 1989). Decorations have not previously been identified as an item retaining personal significance for the resident. The importance of providing locked storage for private papers can not be overlooked.

Display space for personal things can impact other aspects of the facility. Windley and Scheidt (1980) argue that if space to display personal items is provided, offensive behavior would decrease. Millard and Smith (1981) studied the perceptions of the staff when personal items were present. Elderly residents who were surrounded by personal belongings were perceived in a less negative way than the same persons in bare surroundings.

Display space should be more than just a bulletin board. Insulation board can be placed on a larger area or an entire wall and covered with wall carpet or other wall covering which does not show pin marks or nail holes. This allows residents to determine not only what items they wish to display but where they wish to place them.

Shelves should also be available for many items that the resident would like to bring to the nursing home that cannot be attached to a flat surface. These shelves should be adjustable to provide flexibility. Secured cupboards should be provided for the resident who has more valuable possessions (Pastalan & Polakow, 1986).

TERRITORIALITY

Territoriality is often manifested in "ownership" of a particular space or place and often is directed towards a particular chair. Windley and Scheidt (1980) reported Delong observed less territoriality when residents were in private rooms, had space to display personal items and more and smaller spaces for social interaction were provided. Koncelik (1976) reported that less territoriality occurred when the beds in the resident's rooms were placed toe-to-toe rather than both on one wall. In the latter arrangement the person near the window often "owns" the window and the person near the door "owns" the door. Kinney (1987, p. 734) reported "less-alert residents exhibited greater territoriality toward the public spaces than did fully alert residents."

SOCIALIZATION

The importance of designing the environment to facilitate socialization cannot be overemphasized. When the age-related sensory changes, already discussed, occur, the perceptual skills required to communicate in social situations are also affected. Environmental interventions which compensate for these changes will enhance functioning and can improve socialization.

Residents in supportive housing need a variety of social groups. The continuum of socialization needed by each older person ranges from being alone to full assemblage (Snyder, 1978). To provide for each of these social groups unique environmental solutions need to be designed.

Providing spaces for a person to observe and interact with others fosters a sense of social connectedness. Socialization in these informal areas can be fostered through the provision of seating which not only meets the design criteria discussed but also maximizes eye contact and promotes socialization (Sommer, 1970). A sheltered sitting area at the front of a building can foster casual social contact. (See Photograph 3.) A stable glider swing placed in this location can provide opportunities for much needed vestibular and proprioceptive input.

Residents grouped and passively watching is a common occurrence in the long term care facility. This behavior becomes a problem for the staff primarily because spaces have not been created to allow the resident to sit and observe without their presence creating congestion. Because the residents will gather by the nurses station or front door, a specific space must be designed to allow the resident to view these areas of high activity.

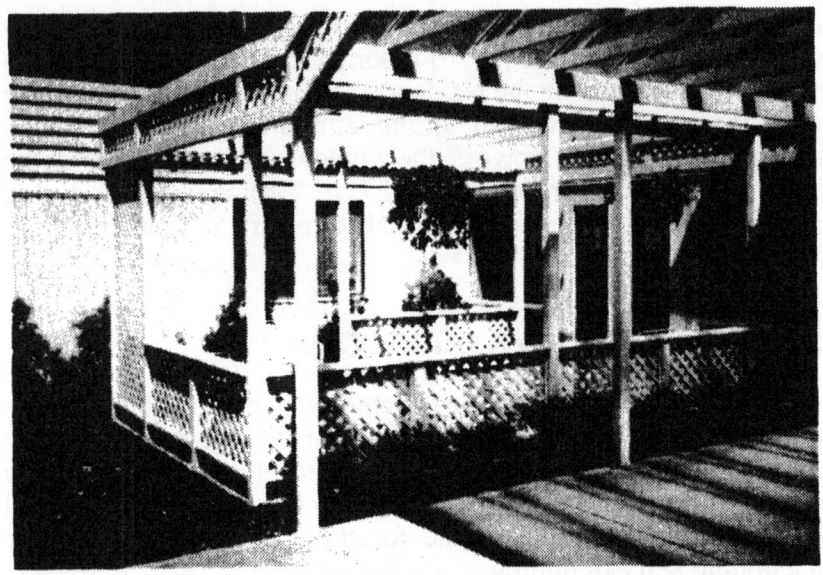

PHOTOGRAPH 3. Sheltered seating area — Assisted Living Project, Portland, OR

In a study of congregate housing, social activity was related to the health status of the individual, the number of available social spaces, and the degree to which residents left doors ajar (Lawton, 1970). Also more socialization occurs when residents are seated at tables (Sommer, 1970) or when residents are in private rather than semi-private rooms (Ittelson, Proshansky and Revin, 1970). Windley and Scheidt (1980) have defined density as the perception of crowding either in absolute numbers or in the proportion of persons to the space. Little is known of the effect of density on an older person's willingness to participate in social programs or whether reduced visual acuity effects a persons perception of crowding.

The goal for social programming and the provision of spaces to socialize is to reduce loneliness but to allow for individual choice. Lounges and other social spaces should be designed for formal arrangements but also have the flexibility to allow the furniture to be moved about by the residents. This adaptability can increase the resident's sense of control.

AESTHETICS

The term aesthetics may conjure up a strictly visual approach to design but fundamental to the definition is the sensual response that is evoked. The term often denotes judgement and good or bad design. An additional approach to aesthetics is a person's perception of quality. Since "there is no agreed upon list of aesthetic principles that adequately assesses the quality of designed environments for the elderly" (Windley & Scheidt, 1980, pg. 413), it is difficult to predict what will be important to the older person. The previous discussion on the meaning of "home" may add insight into this topic. Defining the quality of a space differs between the user and the designer. When one discusses quality, the designer may think of spatial components in terms of rhythm and balance, the user may be more concerned about maintenance and upkeep.

Aesthetics particularly affect the children or friends of the older client. When designing senior housing, and to a lesser degree nursing homes, one is also designing for those who visit the resident. The preferences of visitors must be considered but not to the exclusion of meeting the multiple needs of the resident.

CONCLUSION

As the number of older persons grows, there is an increased awareness among developers, architects, and interior designers that appropriately designed housing will be necessary in the future. Housing that incorporates these environmental attributes and is designed with physical, sensory, social and psychological supports can address previously unmet needs and facilitate "aging in place."

The new Medicare and Medicaid requirements for long-term care facilities, to be implemented some time in 1990, emphasize "environmental quality." The Health Care Financing Administration (HCFA) intends for the new requirements to concentrate on the outcome of resident care. A major change is the focus on the physical environment. "HCFA is seeking a way that nursing facilities can use the available space and the entire environment as a partner in the functional goals of each resident" (Erickson, 1989, pg. 18).

Focus will be placed on environments that encourage social interaction and promote the use of personal possessions (Erickson, 1989). By utilizing the environmental attribute approach, these goals can be accomplished.

Enhancing Independence
in the Home Setting

INTRODUCTION

The trend in long-term health care, both to respond to the preference of older persons (Gallardo & Kirchman, 1987), as well as to attempt to contain costs, is to focus on the home as the center of care. Contrary to popular opinion, care in the home has not been demonstrated to be less expensive than care in a long-term facility. Recent data indicates that community-based long-term care does not save money because rarely do these programs reduce nursing home or hospital care (Weissert, 1989).

However, because an older person's choice is generally to remain in their own home, there is a need to assist the elderly to address age and disability related changes. Typically, community-based assistance is in the form of in-home services; however, the environment itself can be adapted to enhance independence as well. These adaptations can promote independence and relieve the caregiver. A well-designed, appropriately-placed grab bar, that can allow the frail older person to rise alone or with minimum assistance, can eliminate a good deal of physical burden for the caregiver.

Independence must be encouraged in the safest surroundings possible to make the doing of daily tasks easier. Approaching independence from this perspective requires the occupational and physical therapist to step beyond the traditional activities of daily living checklist to develop new ways to assess and evaluate the home. The designer can be called upon to contribute his/her skills to fashion specific products to meet identified needs.

49

SAFETY

When assessing the environment of the older person, safety must be the most important concern. In the United States, where 12% of the population is over 65 years of age, 23,000 persons die each year of accidental death (U.S. Public Health, 1985). Injuries are the sixth leading cause of death in the population of adults 75 and over and falls are the cause of more than two-thirds of the accidental deaths (Azar & Lawton, 1964; Baker & Harvey, 1985).

Seven hundred and fifty thousand persons experience some type of disabling injury each year and are hospitalized an average of 11.7 days for an accident (Parsons & Levy, 1987). In 1981, over 622,000 people were treated in hospital emergency rooms for injuries associated with every day products (U.S. Product Safety Commission, 1985). The chairman of the Special Committee on Aging reports that accidents occurring at home cost $3 billion per year (Molotsky, 1985).

FIRES

Deaths as a result of fires in the home are caused primarily by igniting clothing when smoking or cooking. The mortality rate associated with apparel fires is 49% for persons aged 65 to 80 and 73% for those over 80 (National Safety Council, 1981). One-third of the victims of hot water burns are older persons. Wounds and skin tissue tend to heal more slowly in older persons, hence, burns that do not result in death are especially disabling. Because of a reduced olfactory response, the older person may not be as responsive to leaking gas and the potential for a fire. Gas leak detectors should be placed in senior's homes that have gas appliances.

FALLS

Advanced age is associated with an increased risk of falling. Both the risk of falling and of suffering physical injury increases with age. By the time a person reaches the age of 80, there is a one in three probability of experiencing a damaging fall (Stelman & Worringham, 1985). Incidence rates rise with age and women outrank men in the number of deaths that are caused by falls. This ratio appears to be the same for non-fatal injuries (Melton & Riggs, 1985; Azar & Lawton, 1964).

Studies of falls in the independent elderly have been based upon the response of the older person regarding the conditions that prevailed at the time of the accident. This method does not usually give adequate information about what preceded the accident. Hadley et al. (1985) suggests there is a need for longitudinal studies to assess the functional status of individuals prior to a fall. This study could be designed to provide implicit environmental data.

For every fall that is the underlying cause of death, there are almost 20 falls that result in a fracture of the hip, 84% of these occurring in those over 65 years of age. Hip fracture is the most common diagnosis among all injuries leading to hospital admission in the United States (Baker & Harvey, 1985).

Each hip fracture results in an average of 21 days of short-term hospitalization. Based on hospital and nursing home stays and physicians and surgeons fees as well as indirect cost of lost productivity, new hip fractures in the United States for the year 1980 were estimated to cost 2 billion dollars (Baker & Harvey, 1985). Hip fractures are also a leading cause of disability among the elderly; roughly half of the survivors never recover normal functioning. In the previous figures, follow-up and rehabilitation costs were not included.

The fear of falling creates tremendous anxiety for older persons. "Even if the fall is not serious, the fear of falling is omnipresent and often leads to the refusal to go out, or even go to the bathroom. There is an increase in dependency leading to boredom, depression and, eventually, to becoming bedridden" (Vellas et al., 1987, pg. 192). The family often becomes over-protective and attempts to restrict their older relative's autonomy. In some cases the family's reaction may lead to unnecessary institutionalization.

Contributing Factors to Falls

Non-environmental factors that may contribute to the incidence of falls are postural hypotension, dysequilibrium, decreased vision, decreased proprioception, peripheral neuropathy, reaching, and disorientation. These variables can be a result of the aging process or specific pathophysiology (Parsons & Levy, 1987). In a study by Azar and Lawton (1964) the walking patterns of 2500 elderly women were observed. Twelve percent of these persons were noted to have abnormal gait patterns caused by structural alterations. These women had a narrow walking and standing base, at least a moderate degree of bowing when walking, and altered gait patterns.

Drug usage can be a contributing factor in the incidence of falls. In a study of 196 elderly individuals whose average age was 80, benzodiazepine users were more likely to fall and fall more often, than non-users (Sorock, 1988).

The contribution of gaze stability on spatial orientation has been discussed in an article by Leibowitz and Shupery (1985). They suggest that losses in gaze stability may have important implications for spatial orientation in the elderly and in turn impact upon postural stability.

Postural sway is more prevalent among the elderly person who falls than it is among persons who do not fall (Overstall et al., 1977; Nickens, 1985; Wolfson, 1985). In general, the frequency of falls is related to chronic medical problems. Cardiopulmonary disease and neuromuscular disorders must be considered. Alcohol or antihypertensive medications must be considered as a factor that would effect balance. Anxiety and depression impact not only the individual's fear of falling but effect the person's desire to ambulate and can precipitate the complications of self-restricted activity. Dementia, either multi-infaract or Alzheimer's can predispose an individual to falls (Nickens, 1985).

Most falls are related to physiologic and functional deficits, drugs, or environmental conditions. The prevalence of these causes is difficult to generalize because of the variation between the way in which these factors impact the young-old and those persons over 80 years of age (Hadley et al., 1985; Kennedy & Coppard, 1987).

The reason why the elderly have an increased risk of falling is related to a basic physiological deterioration, compounded by an environment that is not adapted for their physiological conditions. Decreased vision makes it hard to see obstacles as elevation changes, such as the edges of steps or even the chairs in which the older person intends to sit. Poorer reflexes and reduced strength make it difficult to recover balance if a fall is initiated and there is no structural support nearby such as a handrail or stable piece of furniture.

The importance of the sensory and mobility components in the incidence of falls is of primary concern to therapists. Wolfson et al. (1985) have reviewed the complex functions that are effected by both disease and the aging process with respect to the importance of sensory dysfunction in gait and balance problems. Although the effects of age on the integrating structures within the brain have not been defined, it is hypothesized that "abnormalities of gait and balance are produced by dysfunction within the neural mechanism" (Wolfson et al., 1985, p. 650).

Persons who fell frequently, had more gait impairment than non-fallers and there was a two-fold higher vibratory threshold in the lower extremities for fallers than for controls. Neither visual acuity nor vestibular function correlated with falls. The literature indicates that there are decreases in proprioception and touch sensitivity but these were not examined in this study. The most dramatic results were a 10-fold decrease in strength and speed observed in ankle dorsiflexors of fallers. This deficit makes it difficult for the person falling to rapidly adjust the center of gravity to prevent falls (Wolfson et al., 1985).

Environmental Factors Relating to Falls

Because the fall behavior and the environment are inseparable, the focus on injury prevention must not concentrate on the individual alone but also on the the environment where the behavior occurs. Maintaining postural orientation, balance and locomotion are dependent on the surrounding environmental surfaces. A clear, firm, even walking path with adequate visual information is required (Owen, 1985). For the older person to obtain this visual information and move through the space, the importance of adequate lighting and good walking surfaces support must be emphasized.

Falls occur in a variety of places. A person may fall down stairs, trip and fall, fall when arising from bed or chair. These falls may be related to quite different functional or environmental causes. There is no typology that indicates which factors most impact which type of falls (Hadley et al., 1985). Interventions for each situation vary since the deficits that impair our ability to regain balance after beginning to slip on a patch of ice are not the same as those that predispose to falling down stairs'' (Hadley et al., 1985).

Since almost everyone has fallen at some time, the elderly who are most at risk for falls need to be identified. A large share of the falls in the elderly occur for a small percentage of individuals (Hadley et al., 1985). Campbell et al. (1981) analyzed the association and investigated the risk factors of physical and social variables with respect to falls. Falls were divided into two types: pattern and occasional. Pattern falls were those which arose from a disorder of balance, postural instability, and/or perception problems in the person and external input had a minimal effect. Occasional falls were those which had arisen under physical conditions that could have precipitated in a fall in anyone. Women who had patterned falls tended to be older and have poorer vision while men had lower systolic blood pressure. The principle 'predictors' of patterned falls in men were functional disability, the need for support services and informal help. In women, the predictors were not only functional disability, need for support services and informal help, but also the use of walking aids.

Assistive devices are often recommended for the person who is susceptible to falls. The contribution walking aids, such as canes, walkers, and wheelchairs play in the incidence of falls was studied. One hundred fifty persons over age 60 who were treated in an emergency room were reviewed retrospectively. For those persons who used walkers, canes and wheelchairs, assistive devices were considered to have contributed to the accident (Waller, 1978).

HOME ENVIRONMENT

The enormous physical, psychological and economic toll taken by injury to the older person has been discussed. Falls among the elderly are caused by hazards in both the external and home environment. Older persons, because of poor health, are more prone to be in their home (Kennedy & Coppard, 1987). Therefore, for this age group, hazards in the familiar but often very dangerous home environment take on greater significance.

Ninety-five percent of all persons over 65, live in their home and 80% of those over 80. The home is the site for 40% of all fatal accidents (Parsons & Levy, 1987; Gray-Vickery, 1984). The prevalence of falls in the home appears to involve one-third of the population over 65. In persons over 80, this figure rises to one-half.

Older women experience significantly more falls than do older men and these women are also more likely to be living alone. The person living independently may be in a single family or multi-family dwelling. The multi-family may include a variety of housing designed for seniors which may or may not be designed to reduce falls. As the older person experiences the normal changes of aging, the home setting that he/she may have lived in for 40 plus years now develops barriers that do not accommodate to the changes of aging.

For the general population, home injury fatalities can be reduced by 40% through improvements in construction materials and design to reduce hazards; the use of smoke detectors, and poisoning and drowning safeguards would save 10,000 lives per year (Center for Disease Control, 1987). The frequency and severity of accidents in the homes of the elderly emphasizes the need for modifications to compensate for the reduced abilities of the older person.

The most common accident sites in the home are the bathroom, bedroom, kitchen and stairs. Due to the fact that *falls*, fires, poisoning, and suffocations may all occur in the bedroom, it is the most hazardous room in the house. The Consumer Product Safety Commission has determined that stairs are the most hazardous product in the home (Archea, 1985). In the bathroom, *falls*, scaldings, electric shock and drowning can occur. The leading accident occurring on the stairs is *falls*. The kitchen is the primary location of non-fatal injuries, primarily cuts, burns, *falls* and poisioning. Since the scope of this paper does not allow for a discussion of each of these concerns and due to the repetition of falls as the possible cause for accidents in each of these spaces, interventions for falls will be focused upon in the remainder of this section.

Falls/Stairs

Total stairway accidents are estimated to run as high as 2 million per year. One in seven persons will have an accident on a stair that will require hospitalization (Asher, 1977). When walking on a level surface a person's walking pattern is dependent primarily on the length of their stride and their speed of movement. Therefore, foot placement is an individual, albeit unconscious, decision. However, in stair usage, one is highly dependent upon the dimensions and conditions of the stairs. Standards for stair risers and treads are based upon a seventeenth century French formula (Archea, 1985).

Descending a stair is usually more hazardous than ascending. In a study of 32,000 stair users (Carsons et al., 1978), it was determined that an individual undergoes an intricate visual and kinesthetic process prior to descending a stairway. People first look directly at the top stair as they approach and then get proprioceptive feedback as they descend the first two or three steps. In the accidents that occurred in this study, the fallers did not visually attend to the top step. Differences also occurred in kinesthetic behavior. Studies that have been conducted on stair accidents and the elderly indicate that vision may be a major factor in vulnerability. Two leading causes of stair accidents are: visual distractions that draw a users attention away from the stair and visual deceptions built into the design of the stair (Archea, 1985). Several suggestions to increase safety on stairs have been included in the Intervention section.

The potential magnitude of the impact of an intervention is well illustrated by the following situations. In the first, not unusual, scenerio:

> Nursing home placement may be eminent for an elderly widow whose speed and range of walking are severely impaired and who can no longer negotiate stairs. Her only bathroom is on the second floor. (Hadley et al., 1985)

Compare the above situation with an actual case in the study that is being conducted on the prototype stairway handrail system illustrated in Photograph 1 (p. 38). This system provides a retractable handrail which becomes literally a stationery walker on the stair.

Mrs. B, a woman of 85 years with extreme kyphosis ambulates with a walker. She has not been able to go up stairs to sleep in her second floor bedroom. She lives in an area where crime is a concern. On hot summer nights she is not at ease sleeping on the first floor with her windows open. The installation of the retractable handrail has allowed her to return to sleeping upstairs.

The introduction of the specially designed rail has provided a means for Mrs. B to remain comfortably in her own home and maintain her independence.

ASSESSMENT OF INDIVIDUAL

Before addressing environmental interventions to reduce accidents any pathology must be considered and appropriate medical interventions taken. An activities of daily living assessment identifying factors that pertain to the individual should be done by a health care professional, preferably an occupational therapist. This assessment would identify age-related changes and life style issues that impact the environment. The assessment may also identify life style patterns affecting safety that needs to be changed, i.e., wearing loose fitting, or slippery surfaced shoes or slippers on the stairs, retrieving items from high places, not turning on lights when getting up at night.

HOME EVALUATION

The next, often overlooked, step is a *thorough* assessment of the home to identify potential environmental problem areas. When doing home evaluations, occupational therapists have used a variety of tools for many years. Making these evaluations available to the older citizen is a more recent development. Today, home evaluations are also available that allow the older person or their family member to do a home-safety check.

A booklet, Housing for the Elderly: A Self-help Guide (Rabizadeh, 1982) was developed to give the elderly knowledge and guidance to evaluate housing on their own. The guide enables an older person to assess current housing and assists them in evaluating potential housing choices.

In order to reach more older people with this type of evaluation, the U.S. Consumer Product Safety Commission (1985) developed a Home Safety Checklist to provide the older home dweller, family member or friend with a method to spot particular home safety hazards. This checklist may be obtained by contacting the U.S. Consumer Products Safety Commission, Washington, D.C. 20207, (800)-638-2772.

A Home Evaluation Checklist and Resource Booklet for the Elderly were developed and produced by UCLA/USC (Pynoos et al., 1987). These not only evaluate particular areas of concern but also, in the resource booklet, provide practical solutions for the identified problems. This booklet includes several catalogs that list products to remedy some of these identified situations.

Although these and other catalogs exist, the variety of the interventions and/or devices may not be known to the older person, family members or others who could be assisting in initiating these changes. The Gadget Book was published in order to "broaden the awareness of the numerous new 'low technology' products that can make everyday tasks easier and to stimulate the imagination to search for gadgets" (LaBuda, 1985, pg. 9).

The Gadget Book lists products that are readily available, are simple to use, relatively low in cost and can provide immediate benefit. It is divided into areas of activity: personal care, home environment, home maintenance, communications, mobility, health care, leisure and recreation. Each section contains the following product information: Purpose, description, approximate cost, and the way to identify to the manufacturer (LaBuda, 1985).

New methods need to be developed to match the compensatory capacity of these and many other interventions with the age-related changes that occur to older persons. First in this list is education of seniors, family, and friends concerning not only the changes that occur as we age but also the numerous adaptations that are available to compensate for these changes. Additional methods need to be developed to link the needs of the older person with these many devices that can compensate for age related changes.

INTERVENTIONS

The use of low technology devices and interventions can reduce the older person's frustration and struggle with daily activities. Products strategically introduced into the environment of the older person can provide that individual with a method to complete daily living tasks more safely and/or easily.

Environmental interventions can reduce the incidence of falls. A sample of these are listed below:

A. Floor Surfaces:

   1. Carpet

     a. Edges should be tacked down
     b. Wall-to-wall
     c. Low pile

   2. Scatter rugs should be discouraged. If they are present:

     a. They should have non-skid backing of one of the following:

       1. Rubberized backing
       2. Double-faced adhesive tape
       3. Stay-put netting

     b. Should not be placed at top or bottom of stairs

   3. Hard floors (wood or vinyl)

     a. Floor surface should provide stability when wet
     b. Non-skid wax should be used
     c. Spills should be cleaned up immediately
     d. Dust, crumbs and other dry contaminates should be removed

   4. Thresholds

     a. Thresholds should be removed or be low and beveled

B. Stairs

   1. "Lip" on tread should not overhang
   2. There should not be loose or uneven stairs
   3. There should not be torn or curled carpet

4. All carpet and nails should be tacked down
5. Carpet should have low pile
6. Wooden stairs should have non-skid rubber or vinyl treads
7. No objects should be placed on stairs even temporarily
8. The edges of the steps should be distinguishable from the remainder of the step. (Ideally this would be marked with paint, but on interior carpeted steps this would rarely be acceptable. An alternative solution is well lighted stairs.)
9. No two dimensional patterns should be used on stair surfaces
10. Outdoor and/or basement steps should be highlighted with paint or non-slip tape
11. One-step elevation changes should be marked or lighted

C. Lighting

   1. Glare

      a. Lighting should not create any glare
      b. No exposed bulbs in ceiling or table lamps. Lamps should be checked from seated position
      c. No direct glare on stairs through a window

   2. Light switch at door before entering the room
   3. Light bulbs are appropriate size and wattage; if correct size is not known, they should be no more than 60 watts
   4. Light switches or outlets

      a. Light switches should be easily accessible
      b. Outlets and/or switches should not be warm or hot to the touch
      c. Switch/outlet plates should be present

   5. Extension cords

      a. Should never cross traffic path
      b. Should not be under furniture legs or carpet

   6. Lamps

      a. Should be difficult to knock over
      b. Consideration should be given to converting a lamp into

one that can be operated by touch only, thus eliminating the need to search for the switch at night.

D. Furniture

1. Furniture arrangement should provide clear traffic path
2. There should be no lightweight unstable furniture
3. Chairs

   a. Chairs should provide good body support to neck and back
   b. Chair arms should extend far enough forward to provide good support when getting in or out.
   c. Circulation should not be cut off behind the knees when both feet are flat on the floor
   d. Drawers/doors should open easily
   e. Drawer pulls should be easy to grasp

4. Telephone

   a. Letters and numbers should be easy to read
   b. Ring should be easily heard by resident
   c. List of emergency telephone numbers beside phone
   d. Phone should be within reach of the floor

E. Kitchen

1. Hot water temperature should not exceed 130 degrees
2. Dials on stove, microwave should be large and easy to read
3. Stepstool should be stable and have an extension that supports balance
4. Sharp knives/utensils should be stored in a separate, safe place
5. Commonly used items should be within easy reach
6. Household cleaners and disinfectants should be stored separately

F. Bathroom

1. Floor surface should provide stability when wet, preferably be rubberized
2. There should be a non-skid mat/surface used

  a. In the tub/shower
  b. On the bathroom floor

3. Overflow drain must be in good working order.
4. Bathroom door should open outward
5. Bathroom door lock should have a safety release
6. Toilet seat should be at a height that allows the person to get up or down easily
7. Grab bars

  a. Should be attached securely to structural wall supports
  b. Should be installed by toilet
  c. Should be located for entering and exiting tub or shower at shower height (about 40" above the floor) or

    (1) A wall mounted, well supported hand-held shower should be installed as well as a:
    (2) Bench, stool or seat in tub

G. Bedroom

1. Height of mattress should allow the person to place both feet on floor when seated on edge of bed
2. A night stand or other storage unit should be accessible from the bed
3. Storage units/dresser should be sturdy enough to act as a support for person when walking
4. Heating pads should have controlled heat
5. Clock

  a. Should have large numerals on contrasting background
  b. Face should be lighted

6. Emergency numbers should be placed near the telephone.

(Kennedy & Coppard, 1987; Pynoos J. et al., 1985; Christenson, 1988; Rabizadeh, 1982; Archea, 1985)

Additional areas that must receive attention are the design of exterior walking surfaces and railings, interior floors, color contrasts, chairs, acoustical products to remove distracting background noise, as well as the utilization of an array of simple inexpensive adaptations that can foster support and create a more secure environment for the older person.

ADAPTABLE HOUSING

An approach that is gaining more acceptance is that of adaptable housing. "Adaptable housing is housing that does not look different from other housing and which has features that in only minutes can be adjusted added or removed as needed to suit the occupant whether they are disabled, older or non-disabled" (Bostrom et al., 1987, pg. 1). The concept of adaptable housing has been in existence for 15 years but only recently has it been expanded into the senior housing market.

Housing for the older person should address the need to provide accessibility when it is necessary for the older person to use a wheelchair. Adaptable housing can be adjusted or adapted without major structural change because wider door widths, ground level entrances, changeable counter and sink heights, knee space under a work surface, have all been incorporated into the original design.

Other potential interventions are those that can be incorporated into the basic design of an environment. These include: non-glare increased lighting, correctly placed handrails and sound absorbing materials.

When independence includes the use of a wheelchair, incorporating these adaptable housing concepts into the design of homes for seniors can allow the older person to remain in their own home.

ASSISTIVE DEVICES

The appearance of the traditional assistive devices, such as grab bars, reachers, raised toilet seats, have caused many older persons to reject their use. The frail elderly individual who has maintained independence rarely thinks of him/herself as disabled and therefore products that are designed and marketed for the disabled population are often not accepted by the elderly even though they would benefit from their use. As the manufacturers of these devices are becoming more aware of the aging market the appearance of these products is changing. With better marketing hopefully their acceptance will follow.

In addition to the rehabilitation-type devices there are many items which have a more universal application, yet, when they are employed by the elderly meet a special need. Examples of these are: cordless phones, motion activated lights, timed outlet controls, step stool with handrail, under cabinet drawers, long handled dust pans, to name only a few.

The benefit of a particular device or intervention is dependent upon the need of the individual. A device that provides convenience for one person may meet a crucial need for another. We are aware that the older hand with accompanying reduced upper arm strength can much more easily use a lever door handle but that opening that same door for the arthritic hand without that door lever may be totally impossible. In rehabilitation these patient specific approaches have been used for many years. Environmental adaptations must be looked at as well. Appropriate lighting for one person may make reading easier, but for the person with low vision that same lighting creates an environment that allows the person to see well enough to move about safely and independently.

SATISFACTION

The elderly person's perception of the appropriateness of a product or change in lifestyle must also be considered if the full benefit of the intervention is to be obtained.

In 1988, through funding from a Small Business Administration Innovation Research grant, a variety of home evaluation checklists were compiled and subdivided to create a very detailed home checklist. The items on this checklist were matched with specific devices and changes to create a data base of interventions that impact the frail elderly. Because of the commercial development of this data base neither it nor the methodology of the study are available at this time (Christenson, 1989). During a pilot study in Phase I, identified interventions and/or devices were obtained and installed in the homes of seven study participants. After the older person had been using the device for at least a month, a satisfaction questionnaire was administered. (Satisfaction questionnaire is included in the Appendix.)

One older gentlemen, who by all criteria fit the category of frail elderly, would have benefited from a raised toilet seat. However, he did not see himself as frail enough to need that device. On the other hand, a woman who had low vision had already unsuccessfully tried magnifiers but when introduced to a lighted magnifying glass was able to regain independence in doing simple tasks requiring visual acuity.

We must raise the consciousness level of the older person, as well as their families and friends, care providers and policy makers to the wide variety of products that can provide the independence and safety that all desire. The design community must be educated about the structural interventions that must be included in the environment of the older home dweller. Designing housing that will adapt to the individual rather than require the person to adapt to the house is a realistic goal for the home of the older person.

Chair Design and Selection
for Older Adults

INTRODUCTION

Many older persons, due to a variety of physical problems ranging from gradual age-related changes to the sudden onset of a hip fracture or CVA, are not able to move easily from place to place. This immobility creates added importance for the design of chairs for those persons who spend long periods of time sitting in the same place. Regnier and Pynoos (1987) reported on one nursing home study that found that the ambulatory person may spend as much as six hours in a chair whereas for the nonambulatory, often restrained, resident that time may be as much as twelve hours.

There are many types of chairs available on the market today. How does a friend, family member, or an institution go about selecting a chair for one person or a number of persons?

Chairs are designed for different uses from eating to relaxing but the primary focus for any chair selection must be to provide the older user:

- Security when entering or exiting
- Comfort when sitting
- Ease when getting in and out

Providing for security, comfort and accessibility increases the older individual's sense of autonomy. The lack of these environmental attributes affects not only safety, comfort and ease of use, but they have a physical and psychosocial impact on the user. A chair "can produce passivity, apathy and dependence or encourage mobility and independence" (Shipley, 1980, p. 860).

In long-term care facilities the number of persons in wheelchairs has increased measureably. The reduction in the number of persons who are able to walk independently is often attributed to the fact that today older persons are admitted to nursing homes sicker than their counterparts a few years ago. The ramifications of these increased admissions of disabled elderly have far-reaching design implications.

In Minnesota, the typical nursing home has a corridor that is 120 feet in length, eight feet wide and, because of fire codes, lacks any type of seating along this distance. In this state, construction regulations for the distance of resident rooms reads as follows "Patient bedrooms shall be located not more than 120 feet from the nurses' station . . ." (p. 93 Minnesota Department of Health 1987). Often when minimums are established, they become maximums, thus this 120 foot length may then be repeated with the dining room or activities room another 120 plus feet away. The frail elderly resident is left with 240 feet or more to negotiate with no place to sit and rest. The only alternative has been for that person to use a wheelchair.

Because of this design factor, wheelchair use in the nursing home has become the norm rather than the exception. Therapists and physicians have cautioned against the wheelchair being used for long-term seating. The outcome of such lengthy sitting can be large gluteal pressure ulcers, painful flexion contractures and often radial nerve paralysis (Hartigan, 1982). When a person must reside in a wheelchair, an appropriate seated positioning system should be designed (Olin, 1987).

In any type of remodeling of a long-term care facility, unique ways to create corridor seating must be explored. In some facilities changing room usage, down-sizing the number of beds, or rearranging the nurses station may allow for the incorporation of corridor seating. In a one-story facility the support columns were located in such a way that an unused sink space in the resident room could be incorporated with the identical space in the adjoining room, the dividing wall removed and this space opened up into corridor seating (see Figure 1). The facility plans to incorporate this redesign into the remodeling program (Kaste, 1989). An additional benefit of this type of remodeling is that these seating areas visually break up the length of the corridor and not only improve the appearance but enhance wayfinding. Nursing home building codes and/or their interpretation vary among states. Due to this variability, in some areas this type of redesign may not be feasible.

Creating open corridor seating does present one problem, how-

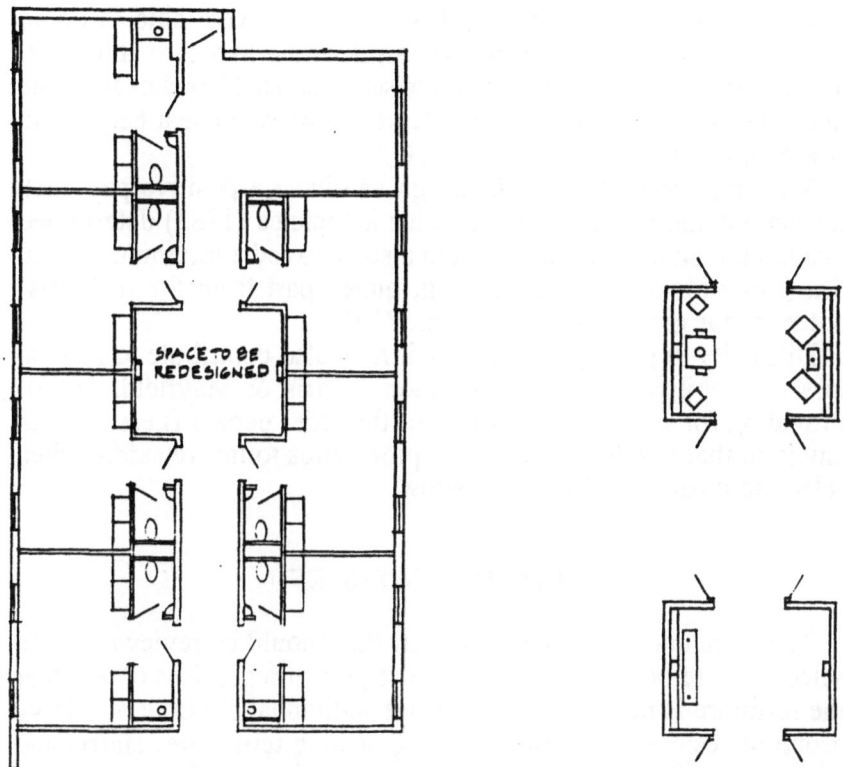

FIGURE 1. Suggested design solutions for corridor seating in a long-term care facility. Small figures represent ways furniture can be arranged in the new space.

ever. Handrails along these sections are eliminated. Ambulatory support must be substituted by the type of furniture that is included in the designed spaces. The weight and stability of this furniture becomes a major factor. Several combinations are possible. These might include a library table with sturdy chairs on each side, two high backed lounge chairs with a table between, or a table for card playing with side chairs. If furniture is not included, handrails should continue in the new space.

The design of the chair itself can have far reaching consequences. In a study of ninety-two residents to determine the effect of lounge chair design on the ability of residents to rise unassisted it was found that seventy-seven percent of the residents who had previously needed assistance to rise from the chair were able to do so independently from a chair that had arms with arm height at least 10 inches above the seat, and where the seat was 16-17 inches from the floor. The study found that the interaction between seat height and arm height was crucial (Finlay et al., 1983).

Selecting the correct chair design can have a positive pay back for the nursing home. Finlay and his associates (1983) determined that in their study "the staff would also be saved a minimum of 300 lifts a day for meals and toileting, quite apart from the residents' potential for greater mobility" (pg. 334).

Difficulty in getting out of a chair may also contribute to general loss of mobility and social isolation (Harris & Mayfield, 1983). Providing for security and safety for the older person is essential in any item that is selected. Specific procedures to insure safety when selecting chairs are discussed below.

CHAIR FEATURES

There are many features of a chair that should be reviewed when selections are being made for an older person regardless of whether the furniture is being selected for one individual at home or a large group of residents in senior housing or long term care. Harris and Mayfield (1983) recommend that the following details be evaluated when selecting a chair for any older individual: Seat height, seat slope, seat depth, clearance under the seat, armrest height to floor at front of chair, armrest height to seat at rear of chair, shape of armrest, backrest slope, backrest shape, upholstery and stability. The basic design of the seat and other safety aspects must also be considered.

Safety and Stability

The older person may substitute the back or arm of the chair for a walker or cane. The chair must provide solid support to allow that individual to move through a space with safety. Chair legs should not be at an angle and extend outward beyond the edge of the seat. This type of design can cause tripping.

The two most common type of chair legs are the traditional leg and a sled-base leg on which a wood piece connects the front and back leg and lies directly against the floor. The sled-base slides more easily over carpet than the traditional chair leg. There have been isolated cases of walkers being caught in the sled base.

Small metal or plastic gliders are often placed by the manufacturer on the bottom of either type leg. The purpose of these gliders is to make the chairs easier to move over the concrete in the factory. If these gliders are left on they actually hinder the movement of the chair on either vinyl flooring or carpet (Christenson, 1989).

Casters have been placed on chairs where carpets are too thick to allow a regular chair to slide easily. Chairs should not have casters nor should thick carpet be installed. To facilitate chair usage, carpets should have a tight density, low loop, no pad and be glued directly to the floor. When this type of carpet is selected, chairs, particularly those that are sled-based, will move quite easily.

In certain cases where a resident is limited to the use of one side of the body, i.e., due to neurological deficits, following a stroke, or after an amputation, he/she may place all of his/her weight on one arm rest. Under these conditions, it is essential the chair does not tip. The stability of the chair and the design of the armrest should be evaluated keeping in mind they may be used for persons with these limitations.

Seat Design

The design of the seat itself is crucial. When a person sits for a long time, it is necessary to change position to relieve pressure on the ischial tuberosities. When the surface on which the non-ambulatory person is sitting is too hard or too much pressure is placed on the bony protuberances, impaired blood supply and inadequate nutrition to the tissue can result in decubitus ulcers (Saxon & Etten, 1987). Bucket or cloth sling-type seats are not acceptable because they do not allow for this needed weight shift. The seat should not "bottom out" so that springs or the wood under-surface can be felt when sat upon for extended periods (Raschko, 1982).

The circulation of blood behind the knee is another concern when evaluating seating. An improperly designed chair cushion can cause compression behind the knee and result in reduced blood circulation to lower extremities (Harris & Mayfield, 1983; Regnier & Pynoos,

1987). Gently curving the front of the cushion can reduce this possibility (Raschko, 1982).

When seating is being selected by a nursing home or senior residence, the staff should test a chair by sitting in it for prolonged periods of time, preferably as long as the resident will sit. The residents should also be given the opportunity to try different designs and their input considered when making final decisions.

The best seat has a flat cushion of firm density that is comfortable during prolonged periods of sitting but allows the occupant to shift their body weight slightly. The seat should prevent the user from hitting or sitting on the hard frame; however, the padding should not be so soft that it is fully compressed by the sitter's body weight. Excessive "give" can cause the sitter to sink down too far into the seat causing problems getting out of the chair. Too little "give" in the cushion will jar both the chair and the sitter when sitting down (Harris & Mayfield, 1983).

Besides meeting the comfort and functional needs of the resident, the special density foam of the cushion should also be inherently fire retardant. Foam is also available which has a fluid barrier, is anti-bacterial, mildew resistant, abrasion resistant and easily cleanable. The latter features add to the cost of the chair but provide a foundation for the application of exciting new upholstry for almost any resident population.

Seat Height

The seat height will be affected by the density of the foam of the cushion. The compressed density of the foam padding must be evaluated when determining the seat height. This will vary slightly depending on the weight of the individual.

The height of the seat should allow the sitter's feet to be supported comfortably, preferably on the floor without pressure occurring under the thigh. The seat height must allow a person to rise easily from the chair. The height for chairs for older women in a nursing home should not exceed 17" because the average height of these persons is 5'2" (Regnier & Pynoos, 1987).

A seat height that causes compression behind the knee or allows the feet to dangle can also reduce blood circulation (Harris & Mayfield, 1983; Regnier & Pynoos, 1987). Body stability is compromised if the height of the seat does not allow the soles of the feet proper contact with the floor surface. When this stability is absent the user cannot change body position and this lack of activity combined with the reduced circulation can cause blood clotting or thrombophlebitis (Panero & Zelnik, 1979).

"Anthropometrically, the popliteal height (the distance taken vertically from the floor to the underside of the portion of the thigh just behind the knee) should be the measurement used as a reference in establishing the proper seat height" (Panero & Zelnik, 1979, p. 63). This ability may be effected by the seat slope and will definitely be influenced by the position of the arms on the chair.

Seat Slope

The slope should be a downward slant from the front edge to the point along which the back of the chair meets the seat. If there is a space between the seat and the chair back, it is at the imaginary point at which these two meet. A steep chair slope can cause difficulty for the person when changing position or rising from the chair. The seat should never slope forward. The slope front to back with the cushion compressed should be between 7-10° (Harris & Mayfield, 1983).

Seat Depth

The depth of the seat is determined by the length of the upper leg and is measured from the rear-most surface of the buttocks to the popliteal space behind the knee (Panero & Zelnik, 1979). If the depth of the seat is too great it will place force on the back of the knee and, as we've already discussed, limit circulation and create potentially dangerous situations.

Another concern for the depth of the seat is that it allow the sitter's lower back to reach and be properly supported by the backrest. Without this stable support greater muscular force is required to maintain equilibrium (Panero & Zelnik, 1979). For the frail elderly, whose strength and stamina are already compromised, the poorly fitting chair compounds their difficulties. If an ideally fitting seat depth is not available, a smaller depth is tolerated better than one which is too great (Panero & Zelnik, 1979; Harris & Mayfield, 1983).

Clearance Under the Seat

To maximize the sitters ability to rise from the chair, the person must be able to place his/her feet beneath the chair and under the body's center of gravity. The chair should not be closed in the front or be designed with a stretcher bar or other piece that would prevent the feet from being placed directly under the seat (Harris & Mayfield, 1983). (See Photographs 1 and 2.) The figures illustrate the foot placement with chairs of two different designs. In a study by Wheeler et al. (1985) it was found the older age group (average age 75) placed their feet farther back under a standard chair when rising than did a younger age group (average age 24).

Armrest Design

The design of the armrest should assist the person to change position with ease and to rest the arms when seated. The armrest will vary depending on the purpose of the chair. If a person is sitting in a particular chair for extended periods the design of that armrest becomes crucial. The armrests must be broad enough to support the lower arm. It should be comfortable and preferably upholstered. If not upholstered the surface should be smooth and all edges should be rounded. Some companies have designed a projection for the hand which extends slightly beyond the front of the seat, to aid the individual to pull themselves forward from the chair. When this protrusion exists, it should be unpadded (Harris & Mayfield, 1983).

Armrest Height to Floor at Front of Chair

Older persons rely on arm muscles as well as leg muscles to come to a standing position. As the older person prepares to come to standing, the arms must be positioned to maximize assistance (Finlay, 1981). The armrest should be basically parallel with the floor with a slope or curve that allows it to be slightly higher at the front than at the back. This position should be high enough to provide support to the sitter in the initial stages of rising from the chair and continue to do so until a stable standing position has been achieved. Due to continual downward thrust exerted on the arms, Finlay

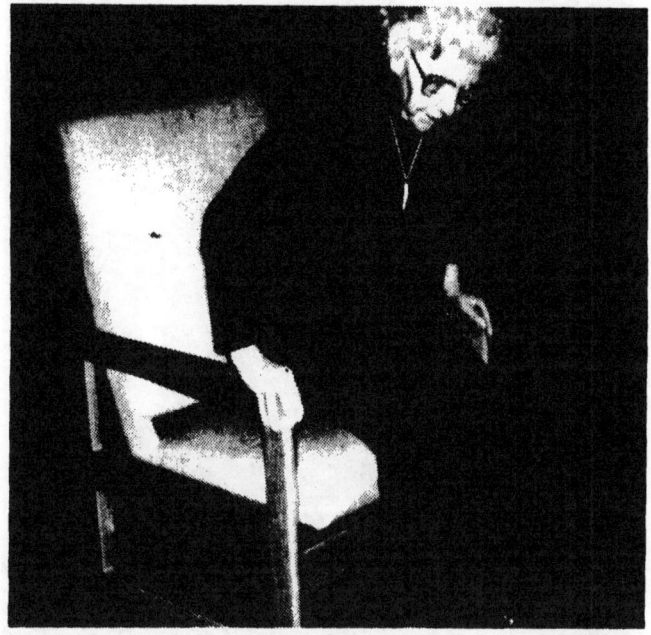

PHOTOGRAPH 1

(1981) demonstrated additional bracing support might be needed where the armrest attaches to the chair.

Armrest Height to Seat at Rear of Chair

The armrest should provide comfortable support to the upper arm when the person is seated. The best design is one that is lower at the back than at the front (Harris & Mayfield, 1983).

Backrest Slope

This slope should allow the sitter to lean back and relax without being so great that it inhibits the person from changing position. The head support region of the backrest should be at less of an angle than the rest of the backrest, so that the sitter gains support for the head without having to excessively extend the neck backwards

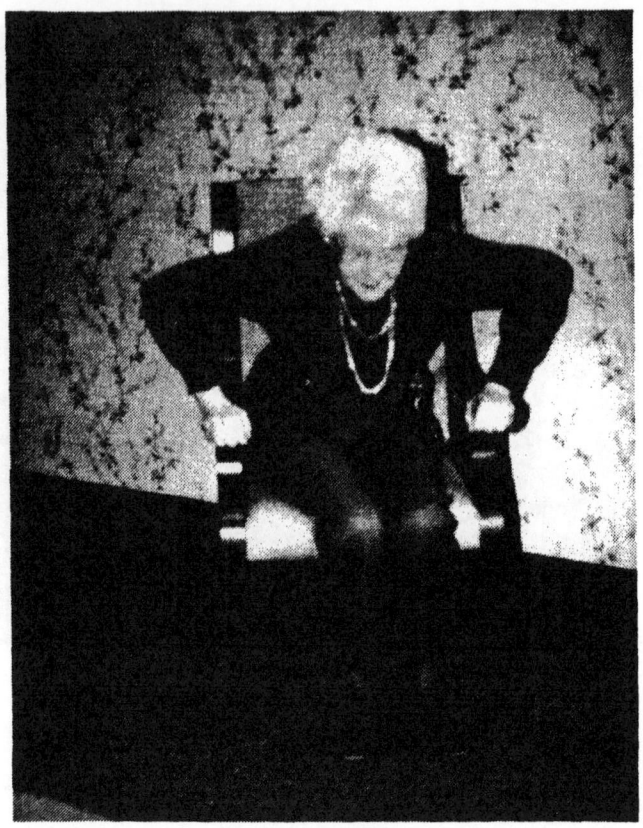

PHOTOGRAPH 2

(Harris & Mayfield, 1983). Care must be taken that the angle does not force the head into flexion.

Backrest Shape

The backrest should provide support for the sitter's lower and upper back regions. The lower, lumbar curve of the backrest should conform with the normal curvature of the back. The person's body should depress the cushioning in the backrest slightly but it should not be so great as to hinder the sitter changing position (Harris & Mayfield, 1983).

Upholstery

There are a variety of materials that may be selected to upholster the chair. In the past, for maintenance reasons, almost all chairs for nursing homes were covered in shiny slick vinyl. Because these materials did not "breath," this upholstery was uncomfortable to sit upon, especially for extended periods of time. New vinyls are now available which do "breath" and are available in a dull finish. These new vinyls come in a variety of softer colors and eliminate the cold clinical appearance.

There are also fabrics that can be used in long term care facilities, even where the resident who is incontinent would be sitting in the chair. This fabric upholstery is velcro attached and, when soiled removed from the chair, cold water washed, line dried and returned to the chair. The cushion is covered with a vapor barrier that prevents moisture from entering the padding. The aesthetic appeal of these fabrics can not be under estimated. Fabrics can also be used in concert with vinyl, e.g., the vinyl can be placed on the seat and the fabric on the back.

Fabric can also be vinylized. This process places a vinyl coat over a fabric and the material can be cleaned the same as one would clean regular vinyl. The advantages to this fabric treatment is that bright prints and more residential materials can be incorporated into the environment. The disadvantage is that this finish does not "breath" and should not be used on pieces that provide prolonged seating. This fabric is often used quite effectively for dining room chairs.

TYPES OF CHAIRS

Lounge Chairs

This chair is used for extensive periods of sitting. It is the type found in lounge spaces and usually, a slightly scaled down model, in the resident room. The chair provides head and neck as well as back support and is designed for seating for extensive time periods.

Side Chairs

This chair is lighter and used for seating in dining room, library, or for card playing, and activities. This chair is used for seating for shorter periods of time.

Sofas/Couches

In lounge space, furniture that provides seating for more than one person is often desirable. This type may be selected for appearance as well as economy of space. These pieces should be limited to seating for two persons. When three-seater units are placed in areas used by the elderly, the center portion, obviously, is left without arms, thus creating a space from which rising is next to impossible. Firm seat cushions and seat height are equally as important for these two-seater pieces as they are for the single chair.

Rocking Chairs

The vestibular input provided by rocking can not be overlooked. Since level of stimulation of this sensory system varies from individual to individual, the rocking chair provides an excellent self-directed modality.

Getting in and out of a rocking chair that is used by seniors must be given utmost consideration. Because of the instability of the traditional rocking chair, other alternatives should be looked for. Some companies have incorporated a stop on the bottom of the rocker so that when the chair comes all the way forward, a stable base is formed for exiting.

Rocking chairs that are specially designed for use in health care settings usually have a rocker or glider mechanism upon which the individual sits. The arms are part of a stable frame. This arrangement provides a stable surface for the older person to grasp when getting in or out of the chair.

Another company utilizes a dynamic seating design. Although this chair may not be designed primarily as a rocking chair, it does provide a slight rocking motion. This chair is covered with a mesh-like seat and back that keeps the user cool and dry.

Recliners/Contour Chairs

Seniors have been enticed by advertising for seat-lift recliners. This type of chair provides automatic rising assistance to an individual. The advantages versus the cost of this type of chair are questionable.

Contour chairs provide seating in a semi-reclining position. They are very difficult to get in and out of. There may be instances, for the non-independent individual that they might be helpful; for example, in a hospice unit.

Stacking Chairs

Side chairs are often used where space economy is a must. One can stack these chairs when not in use and, when space is limited, provide other activities in the area. The disadvantage is an integral part of the design, that is, to allow stacking, the arms must project outward. This design feature can create stability problems. If all of an individual's weight is placed on one side, tipping is quite possible.

Patio Furniture

All of the considerations listed above should be incorporated into the selection of outdoor furniture. There are several inexpensive attractive outdoor chairs on the market; however, most of these are lightweight and unstable. Well designed patio furniture can increase the use of the space. Single moveable chairs allow for more flexibility to adapt to weather conditions and the group size than does fixed furniture. Seating surfaces should be wood or vinyl cushioned. Hard, cold surfaces such as concrete should not be used (Carstens, 1985).

Geri-Chairs

The geriatric wheelchair was designed to provide additional physical support for the frail individual but it has been used as a restraint with little consideration for the psychological effect the chair may have on the older individual. The high backrest restricts vision and the overall increased size of the chair decreases the spaces in which it can be placed. The chair "resident" usually is restricted to the periphery of any social space. Hiatt (1975) has pointed out that "a device that isolates the individual is at odds with the stated goals of nursing home care" (p. 19).

Toilet Seat

A toilet seat is crucial to maintaining continence, Brink (1985) recommends toilet seat height be at conventional chair heights. Toilet fixtures are available in a variety of heights. The 17 1/2" to 18" height should be installed for use by the older person. A 20" "accessible" height is available but this stool is too high to allow for proper elimination.

Bed Height

Since most older persons fall in the bedroom (Tideiksaar, 1988), the height of the bed must be considered in any discussion on seating height. For the older person of average height, a safe bed height is about 18" from the top of the mattress to the floor. A mattress and padding is usually about 4" so a bed frame height should measure about 14" from the floor. Allowances must be made for those persons who are extremely short or tall.

CHOOSING A CHAIR FOR A GROUP OF PEOPLE

In an establishment such as a retirement center, day care center, or a long-term care center, where seating is so crucial, selecting *a chair* that will be comfortable for all persons in a group is an impossible task. Each chair must cater to a number of users. A limited range of chairs must be selected which will adequately accommodate a range of people. A method is needed to assist in determining this range. Chairs must accommodate a range of sizes and yet quantity purchases dictate that the number of sizes that are selected must be limited.

Based on extensive ergonomics testing at the Institute for Consumer Ergonomics, University of Technology in Loughborough, England, a formula for chairs selection was established (Harris & Mayfield, 1983) that will accommodate the comfort of 90% of the residents. This formula gives a facility direction to order chairs of the same style but in three different dimensions: a low narrow, an intermediate wide or intermediate narrow and a high wide. The choice of which type of intermediate chair to buy would be based on the residents being served. In a mostly male population the intermediate wide would probably be selected, with a facility with more women, the intermediate narrow would probably be a better selection.

An even more sophisticated selection can be made that will accommodate 92% of the population. The latter requires the purchase of five chair sizes. Without changing the basic chair sizes, this percentage may be improved to 94% by the addition of a footrest and improvement of the headrest region.

The following example illustrates how, when using the formula, the adequate number of three different sized chairs can be determined.

If 30 chairs are desired, using chair sizes A, C, and E from Table B or C, the sum of the ratio is 3.6 (1 + 1.3 + 1.3), as found in Table A.

The number of chair size A needing to be purchased is, therefore, the total number of chairs divided by the sum of the ratios, multiplied by the ratio for chair size A, i.e.,

$$\frac{30}{3.6} \text{ x } 1 = 8.3, \text{ i.e., 8 chairs}$$

Similarly for both chair sizes C and E,

$$\frac{30}{3.6} \text{ x } 1.3 = 10.8, \text{ i.e., 11 chairs}$$

Thus if a total of 30 chairs are needed there should be:

    8 chairs of Size A
    11 chairs of Size B or C
    11 chairs of Size E

Table A's selection ratio is based on this formula. Tables B and C include approximate chair size recommendations. Measurements are in inches. A range of sizes is given because consensus among referenced material did not occur (Harris & Mayfield, 1983; Raschko, 1982; Finlay et al., 1983; Wheeler et al., 1985; Koncelik, 1976; Panero & Zelnik, 1979).

TABLE A. Selection Ratios

Ratios based upon:	1	1.3	1.3	1.1	1.3	% of persons accommodated in selection
No. of chairs to be selected						
Five	X	X	X	X	X	92%
Four	X	X	X		X	91%
Four	X	X		X	X	91%
Four	X		X	X	X	91%
Three	X		X		X	90%
Three	X				X	90%

TABLE B. Approximate Lounge Chair Size Recommendations

Dimensions in inches	A Low Narrow	B Inter- mediate Narrow	C Inter- mediate Wide	D High Narrow	E High Wide
Seat Height	15-16	16-17	16-17	17-18	17-18
Seat Depth	18	18	18	19	19
Seat Width	17-20	17-20	18-22	17-20	18-22
Approx. back rest height	27-31	27-31	31-34	27-31	31-34
Armrest Height to seat	7-9	8-10	8-10	8-10	8-10
Armrest Length	18	18	20	18	20
Armrest Height to floor at front	24-25	25-26	25-26	27-28	27-28

Seat slope
compressed $7 - 10°$ for all sizes

TABLE C. Approximate Side Chair Size Recommendations

SIDE CHAIR Dimensions in inches	A Low Narrow	B Inter-mediate Narrow	C Inter-mediate Wide	D High Narrow	E High Wide
Seat Height	15-16	16-17	16-17	18-20	18-20
Seat Depth	16	16	16-17	16	16-17
Seat Width	17	17	18-21	17	18-21
Armrest Height to seat	7-8	8-10	8-10	8-10	8-10
Armrest Length	18	18	20	18	20
Armrest Height to floor at front	26	27	27	28	28

Redesigning the Long-Term Care Facility

Margaret A. Christenson, MPH, OTR
Deon Gieneart, BS

INTRODUCTION

A clearer understanding of age-related sensory changes has prompted a closer examination of the function of present day long-term care facilities. Technological advances in forms such as carpeting, wall covering, and lighting; insights into the psychological and physiological impact of the designed environment; and the sobering demographic reality of an aging population point to a new approach.

The original concept of long-term care facilities was based on a medical model which was developed to care for the seriously ill individual with one primary diagnosis. Many older persons have more than one chronic condition, however, and are not acutely ill. The very old (85+) are likely to be frail and have multiple disabling conditions. Compounding the problem are adult children who are themselves approaching an age where physical and financial resources are limited. Often, long-term care facilities are the only alternatives available to the frail elderly.

Administrators, architects and designers are challenged to redesign long-term care facilities to compensate for age-related changes. To design a nursing "home" instead of a hospital, the long-term care facility must differ from the medical model that has evolved since the founding of the first hospitals in America.

The author would like to extend special thanks to Deon Gieneart, graduate student, Mankato State University, for her assistance in compiling the data from the six long-term care facilities.

HISTORICAL PERSPECTIVE

To understand the present day nursing home it is helpful to review the historical development of hospitals. In 1752 Dr. Thomas Bond and his friend Benjamin Franklin opened the Pennsylvania Hospital in Philadelphia, devoted solely to the care of the ill (Millenson, 1988). Designed for those who had once earned an "honest living," but were elderly, injured (or their widows), the "worthy poor" were admitted to the first hospitals. The "unworthy poor" were sent to almshouses which originally housed orphans and criminals as well as the poor, aged, insane and disreputable. The affluent were treated at home.

As the middle class grew, so did the demand and willingness to pay for better care. The discovery of ether and sterilization techniques cemented the idea that hospitals were the premium site for people of all social classes to obtain the maximum quality medical care. The Civil War, growth of cities to accommodate the huge influx of immigrants, and the westward migration promoted hospital construction. Two World Wars, economic expansion, further scientific and technological advances brought healthcare to an unprecedented and sophisticated system.

With the end of World War II, Congress, acting on a shortage of hospital beds, passed the Hospital Survey and Construction Act, known as the Hill-Burton Act. The original law was amended to include the expansion of hospitals, nursing homes, rehabilitation facilities and diagnostic and treatment centers. In the mid-1960s, answering the pressing needs of the aged and indigent, Congress established Medicare and Medicaid (Millenson, 1988). Churches answered the call for help to house elderly in nursing homes, and hospitals extended their mission as well. These driving forces were behind the proliferation of nursing homes.

The changes in healthcare delivery, coupled with what we have learned about age-related changes, are cause to reexamine the original concept of nursing home design. It has become evident that the acute care medical model is not functional for the long-term care geriatric patient. Efforts to provide a home-like, safe environment that enhances the dignity of the individual are under way not only in new construction but in the redesign of existing long-term care facilities.

If the present long-term care facilities are to be made more home-like, however, major adaptations of the medical model are required. Although the site and the size of facilities will vary, the components of the settings will be comparable. Each must find design solutions for lighting, floor and wall covering, finishes, fixtures and furnishings. If the facility has more than one floor, additional cueing of elevators will be indicated. Compensations for direct glare, acoustical considerations, accessibility, codes and standards will be similar.

In this section the environmental concerns found during consultations to six Minnesota long-term care facilities will be discussed. Many of the facilities exhibited similar situations. These conditions ranged from reduced sense of privacy and control of the personal environment to major safety factors. Each facility also presented unique design considerations. This section will examine some of the environmental conditions occurring in these facilities and describe recommendations that were proposed to compensate for these circumstances.

Rationale for many of these suggestions is included. The additional background for this rationale is included in other sections in this publication. This is covered in the sections on sensory changes in the older person and the attributes the environment provides.

LIGHTING

Lighting can enhance or hamper the comfort and safety of the elderly person. Problems are created when there is too little light or too much. The latter often results in glare. In the long-term care facility, too little light may be the result of excessive energy conservation. It is quite common in nursing home corridors to turn out every other light. This creates a combination of the pooling of light and extreme shadow which can be misinterpreted as steps. Glare is so pervasive a challenge that it extends far beyond the subject of illumination and into nearly every aspect of living in the long-term care facility. For example, shiny floors, the pride of the housekeeping department, can be a major safety hazard because of glare.

There are two types of overhead lighting—indirect and direct. Direct lighting is usually incandescent. The typical incandescent lamp has a wire filament, is pear-shaped and screws into a socket. Incandescent lighting may or may not create glare depending on the placement and the fixture. Indirect lighting eliminates glare, creates even lighting and is usually fluorescent. Light from a fluorescent lamp is produced when electricity passes through phosphors within the bulb. Typically, fluorescent bulbs are long and tubular (Nuckolls, 1976). Fluorescent lighting uses much less electricity than an incandescent lamp to produce the same amount of light. A 40 watt fluorescent bulb gives as much light as a 150 watt incandescent bulb (Paulson, 1982). Since these bulbs are more cost effective they are often used in the nursing home.

Fluorescent lighting must be selected carefully and ballasts checked to be sure flickering is minimized. Problems with the use of fluorescent lighting for the elderly usually relate to flickering of the light or the color of the bulb. There are two types of fluorescent light bulbs used in the long-term care facility, warm and cool white. Cool white bulbs have a yellowish-green tone and warm white bulbs give a softer tint to skin tones and to the room in general. Cool whites tend to be installed more often than warm whites because the purchasing agent may not be aware that there are alternatives. The interior designer needs to be advised as to the color bulbs to be used because the quality of the lighting affects design choices.

Flickering is caused by either bulbs ready to burn-out or ballasts that need replacing. Flickering can be minimized if ballasts are checked carefully and a routine bulb replacement schedule is used.

The traditional long tubular bulb is usually installed in the center of the ceiling parallel with the wall. Fixtures for this lighting should have parabolic lenses (egg-crate type) so that the direct light source is obscured and there is no glare.

Incandescent light in the ceiling is usually placed in a can fixture. Although this lighting adds warmth and style, it may create shadows and light pools and often cannot provide adequate illumination. A smaller fluorescent light bulb has been developed that can be placed in a deep ceiling fixture. The light is maximized by a highly reflective surface within the can. With the introduction of these bulbs, illumination levels can be increased markedly. Since low light levels in corridors are a very common problem, utilization of this type of fluorescent lighting has the potential of markedly improving corridor lighting in long-term care facilities that are being redesigned.

Minimal corridor lighting for nursing homes is listed at "10 footcandles" (Minnesota Dept of Health, 1987, pg. 127). The Illumination Engineering Society recommends "20 footcandles in corridors for persons over age 55" (Kaufman, 1981, pp. 2-5). Since the nursing home population is 80 plus and they require 3 times the light of a twenty-year-old (Christenson, 1988), these minimums are not adequate. New standards for nursing home lighting need to be established.

Supplemental task lighting in the form of desk lamps, table lamps by chairs for reading or close work and lighting for specific activities is essential for persons at any age. Sometimes, in the nursing home, providing this additional lighting is overlooked. Whereas corridor lighting might require 30-40 footcandles, a table lamp for reading might require anywhere from 50 to 100 footcandles depending on the individual user (Raschko, 1982). Recessed lumination, ceiling-mounted, can be installed over a game table. Track lighting in lounge spaces can be directed on seating groups. Desk lamps for writing, typing and hobbies, will not only enhance vision, but can be decorative and less institutional.

Examples of Lighting Improvements

In one Minnesota nursing home, the overriding issue was lighting, particularly in the corridors. Several suggestions were made to alleviate this problem. The first was the use of indirect lighting recessed in the suspended ceiling on each side of the corridor. This type of modification is dependent upon the location of pipes, heat ducts, and wires under the suspended ceiling.

A second solution to reduce glare was to install a wall-mounted valance that concealed the source of light and spread it indirectly up on the ceiling. The valance must be opaque to eliminate direct glare. This lighting might be more economical to install since some wiring already existed to accent lights. Additional information on the extent of additional wiring was not available at the time of the consultation. Creating even lighting would be more difficult with valance lighting since wall-mounted fixtures would be located between doors and continuous lighting would not be possible.

Other possibilities were to retain the current light placement and to use parabolic louvers. If the smaller fluorescent lights described above were used a new can-type receptacle would have to be installed.

This facility had accent lights with opaque bulbs which created direct glare. Discussion with the staff indicated a desire to retain some accent lighting. The necessity to create a non-glare source was discussed with the staff. Suggestions included brass accent lights that would provide indirect light.

WINDOW TREATMENT

The need for window treatments that would meet the visual needs of the residents played a large role in these consultations. Design solutions varied and included using a mylar film which either adheres directly to the window, or is in the form of pull down shades; blinds—vertical or horizontal; pleated polyester shades; draperies, or a combination of several treatments.

Recommendations were based on the following considerations. Mylar film, adhered directly on the window, would control the dazzling sunlight, but would also make a gloomy day seem even grayer. On the other hand, pleated shades, which give a softening, more residential effect, have no room-darkening capability. Vertical blinds are easily moved to control for sunlight and privacy and can be fitted with wall covering to coordinate with other furnishings, however, they may produce a distracting sound if used on open windows or near air ducts. Mini-blinds control for sunlight quite well, but are more difficult to clean. All elements—exposure to sunlight, proximity to ducts, maintenance, need for privacy and room-darkening capability—were assessed before making recommendations.

One facility commanding a panoramic view contained a variety of windows which called for different solutions. The windows, other than those in the chapel and dining room, divided into two basic designs: casement, with six panes of glass on the bottom and six on top; and another larger type with a single pane in the center and smaller casement windows on each side.

Direct glare was a problem at most of the windows in this facility. Glare-reducing window treatment was recommended for the windows on the east, west and south. This facility was assessed during the summer. Because of indirect glare from the snow in the winter, glare might also be a problem on the north.

The dining room windows presented some unique challenges because they extended two stories toward a high ceiling. Direct glare existed through the upper half-round portion of the window. This glare was most noticeable in the balcony, an area where the more confused residents ate. The upper portion of the window could be treated with adhered window film or shirred casement window treatment. Vertical blinds, properly fire-rated, should be installed on the long vertical part of the windows.

For the side casement windows with large center panes, the solutions could be either vertical blinds or mylar pull-down film plus draperies. The primary recommendation was to use the mylar shades and to add full, solid color drapery with tie-backs on each side and a valance at the top of the window.

The solutions for the multi-paned casement windows depended upon the use of the rooms they served. Drapery/shade or sheer combinations would block glare but when closed eliminate the view. Translucent permanently-pleated polyester shades eliminate glare while retaining the view. The pleated shades also reduce window heat loss in the winter and reflect the sun's light and heat in the summer, however, they have no room-darkening capabilities. In areas where room darkening is necessary, e.g., the showing of movies, room-darkening drapery will be necessary. Where privacy is a concern in resident rooms, draperies should be added. To soften appearances in any of these rooms, a valence could be added to the windows.

CEILINGS

Acoustical tile, used in suspended ceilings, was one of the primary sound attenuating materials in the nursing homes observed. However, tiles especially designed to absorb sound in the frequency range where speech is most intelligible, did not seem to be installed. In facilities that were replacing ceiling tile, it was recommended these specially designed tiles be selected. Special consideration was given to corridors, where the need for better speech discrimination and reduction of noises created by staff, residents and equipment, was a particular concern.

Ceiling fans are a popular solution to air circulation. They may be noisy, however, and if the moving fan blades are in the person's line of peripheral vision, they can cause distraction. This irritation is compounded if the blades contrast in color with the ceiling. In this instance, the disoriented person will become increasingly confused.

In one nursing home where dark ceiling fan blades revolved against a white plastered ceiling, the recommendation was to replace the blades with some the same color as the ceiling. It was also suggested that acoustical tile be installed to reduce the noise level produced by the fan.

WALL COVERINGS

The type and amount of pattern in a wall covering is an important factor when selecting material which will serve the needs of staff and residents in a long-term care setting. Ease of maintenance is also a major factor and few patterned wall coverings are available in the quality that is needed to withstand the wear and tear of a nursing home. Wall coverings must be in compliance with the fire code.

Selected companies specialize in durable, patterned wall covering. If the residents are alert many patterns may be quite acceptable. While patterns may first appear to convey a more residential feeling, caution must be taken when selecting wall covering for the person with dementia. When dementia is compounded by visual deficits, patterns can appear as frightening forms, such as bugs or worms.

Wall coverings do more than provide color, texture and pattern in a nursing home. The color and design of the wall covering can serve as valuable landmarks. The wall covering also acts as a backdrop for other landmarks and signs.

LANDMARKS

Cues such as landmarks and signs are those items in the environment that facilitate orientation and way finding. The corridors in senior housing or a long-term care facility often lack these cues. The more confused a person becomes the more landmarks or cues are needed to select, from whatever sensory and cognitive ability he or she has remaining, an environment that has meaning.

Landmarks are cues such as specific pictures or objects that help one establish where one is in a particular space. The utilization of bold prints or pictures at specific points can help orient residents, staff and visitors in a facility. Often the importance of these landmarks has been overlooked because wayfinding is not emphasized in the architectural design and the "art budget" is looked at from aesthetics only. Guidelines for selecting landmarks and signage are included in the Appendix.

The nursing home unit of one rural hospital lent itself easily to use of color for orientation. The recommendations for the three principle corridors with adjacent resident rooms and community spaces were to use three major color schemes; red tones in one corridor, yellows in another, and to tie in with the rest of the hospital design, blue tones in the third. The suggestions included carrying out the theme incorporating the recommendation on landmarks in the guidelines.

Designing a nursing home can be facilitated by beginning with a theme. Often the artwork can carry out the theme effectively and serve as a cue for the residents as well. Every corridor should have its unique quality and identity using distinctive subjects, colors and shapes. Pictures, wall hangings and/or other artifacts, perhaps chosen by a resident/staff council, which have realistic patterns and subject matter to which the residents can relate, can be particularly pleasing and useful.

In one Northwestern Minnesota nursing home, themes were selected that tied in with the surrounding geographic area. Themes included farming, lakes, fishing, hunting and other scenes familiar to the residents. It was recommended that these themes be incorporated into the artwork in corridors, i.e., a nautical theme with pictures and wall hangings of boats and fishing and a farming theme with pictures of farm equipment and animals raised on the farms.

The majority of pictures selected for nursing homes and/or senior housing are prints of pictures or photographs. Photographs usually have muted tones and subtle changes. It may be very difficult for the resident with reduced visual acuity, color discrimination and/or depth perception deficits to discriminate details. The reproduction of many pictures is of poor quality resulting in a picture which is faded and difficult for the resident to see.

Another factor when selecting artwork for a long-term care facility is the size of the wall space. In an attempt to make a nursing home "homelike," a common design error is made by using items that are appropriate for a home on the walls of a corridor. This usually does not work because these items are out of scale. A long hallway requires a large picture or other type of wall treatment that is in scale with the length of the corridor. Small pictures on long walls tend to emphasize the length. Groupings of small pictures with like subjects, style or color can serve the same purpose as one large painting.

Fabric art products and large posters are dramatic and relatively inexpensive. Since photographic studios are usually able to do posters for a minimal cost, changing wall decor occasionally can be feasible. Corridors can be transformed into art galleries with pictures selected by the resident's council. This may be a permanent or rotating collection, depending upon the orientation level of the residents. The changing of landmarks should only be considered for the alert residents because of the importance of cues.

In another nursing home in a small Minnesota farming community, contact prior to the consultation had been made with one of the key staff persons. She had implemented the following ideas. In this facility of Norwegian, Swedish and German heritage, a delightful design solution centered around the ethnic backgrounds of the residents. Wooden shelves, decorated with the colorful Norwegian folk art of Rosemaling contained dried flowers and other items meaningful to the residents. In addition to being cheerful and beautiful, the designs represented important reminders of the cultural, educational and occupational heritage of the people living there.

Other design solutions that included art in the same nursing facility were use of quilts as wall-hangings and display cases to hold "old country" items as reminders of resident's ethnic background. Farm kitchen items, particularly from the 1920s and 1930s might be a source of pleasure to those men and women who came from farm backgrounds.

In a therapeutic park designed for the "mentally frail" artifacts were displayed. Included were a one-hundred-year-old plow and an old-fashioned water pump (Carstens, 1985). If this is an area used by the person with dementia, the resident should be able to actually pump water. This could be done with a buried hose with turn-off controls at the main building.

FLOOR COVERING

Floor covering competed with lighting as a major issue in the design of the nursing homes in these consultations — especially in corridors. The alternatives for floor covering were shared with these facilities.

The major options in floor coverings are either a hard surface: vinyl, or a soft surface: carpet. Vinyl comes in different types of material — composition tile and sheet vinyl. There are two types of sheet vinyl used in nursing homes; one is residential, that does not have to be waxed but may lack the ability to tolerate nursing home use. The other is a commercial grade. Because of the wear and tear that occurs in a nursing home setting, commercial sheet vinyl manufacturers recommend the waxing of that surface. Therefore, even though one installs sheet vinyl, rather than composition tile, the indirect glare problem is not eliminated.

The other alternative is carpet. There are many pros and cons raised about using carpet in a nursing home. First and foremost among staff concerns is odor. If an incontinent resident urinates on the floor of vinyl composition tile or sheet vinyl, the natural response is to be concerned about someone slipping and falling. As a result, the wet spot gets immediate attention. When the floor surface is carpet, there is not the same anxiety about safety and therefore these stains are not always cared for as rapidly as they would be on a hard surface. With any type of carpet the staff should have an emergency stain removal kit with solutions for general categories of stains at their disposal for prompt usage.

While stains and odor are still valid considerations, the advent of solution-dyed, rather than yarn-dyed, fibers has produced a carpet in which the color permeates all the way through the fiber, thus, even when a stain of some magnitude occurs, it can be removed with full strength bleach. (Methods for stain removal are included in the Appendix.) Lingering odor in a carpet may be due to moisture reaching and penetrating the floor surface. Carpet with a special liquid-barrier backing prevents this type of penetration.

The carpet should contrast in color with the wall. Contrast will help the resident with reduced depth perception to define the boundary between wall and floor.

One further objection to carpeting in nursing homes is that the additional amount of friction and resistance will make propelling wheelchairs and/or carts more difficult. The type and weave of the carpet selected become crucial in addressing this issue but dense, low-looped pile which is very tightly woven will provide a surface over which most individuals can push a wheelchair. Changes in floor covering may require a short period of adjustment. Also, additional lubrication of the wheelchair or equipment will help all but a small percentage of the frail elderly residents with weak upper extremities adjust to carpeted surfaces.

On the plus side, carpet has several qualities that hard surface flooring does not have. The three major benefits of carpet are: reduction of glare, absorption of sound, and creation of a more secure environment. In addition, the aesthetic impact of a more residential atmosphere cannot be overlooked in what is to be a home, not a hospital.

FURNISHINGS AND FIXTURES

The subject of seating — side chairs, lounge chairs, two-seater sofas, patio furniture-has been addressed in depth in another section. There are compelling reasons for close attention to specifications for seating for the elderly and the long-term care facilities studied here had a variety of specific unanswered needs.

Along with chairs, tables which need to be suited to ambulatory residents but often must be wheelchair accessible, present design problems. In addition, occasional tables, such as coffee tables, are a safety hazard. The best general solution is to remove all low tables to allow for resident's visual and/or balance problems. The remaining tables, either pedestal or with legs, need to be very stable.

Pedestal tables allow easier accessibility by wheelchair users, but when an ambulatory person rests his/her weight upon them they can tip more easily than tables with legs. The larger the diameter, the heavier the pedestal base must be in order to prevent tipping. These heavier bases make it difficult for the maintenance staff to move them. There are tilt-type pedestal tables which allow for flexible space usage since they occupy less than 10 percent of the original usable space. There must be 29 inches of clearance under the table top for wheelchair accessibility (AOTA, 1983). A table at this height is uncomfortable for the ambulatory resident when seated. If the seat of the chair is higher from the floor, the ambulatory resident's feet will dangle. Consideration should be given to an adjustable-height table to accommodate both wheelchair and ambulatory residents.

Tables with legs, usually square, are more stable and less space-demanding, but more difficult for the person in the wheelchair to negotiate. Square tables can be put in a series to form long tables, a practical consideration for multi-purpose rooms. Furniture legs that extend past the line of the edge of the table can cause a tripping hazard. The color of the seat cushion of chairs selected for dining rooms or lounges should contrast in color with the floor covering so it is distinguishable by people with sight disabilities (Reznikoff, 1979).

One facility had attempted to solve the problem of floor space by using a table designed to be stored at ceiling height when not in use. When lowered to the table height position, metal girders support it from the ceiling. Although this table is quite stable and allows for wheelchair access, the unusual arrangement of the metal girders hamper visual contact and reduce the amount of socialization that could be feasible at the table.

HARDWARE

General specifications for interior accessibility include providing hardware, both latching and nonlatching, operable with a single hand that does not require wrist action or fine finger manipulation (Reznikoff, 1979). Other suggestions for hardware include: provision of texture on door hardware for identification and use of lever handles on all side-hung latched doors.

OUTDOOR SPACES

The design of outdoor areas often does not respond to the special needs and requirements of the elderly. A place for resident participation in nature is an important consideration. Walkways can provide a series of longer and shorter routes and because of the older person's sensitivity to glare, direct viewing areas in shade are important. Gates should be de-emphasized and, if a fence is necessary, it should be as unobtrusive as possible.

A suggestion to reduce the visibility of a particularly noticeable chain link fence, in one facility, was to paint it green and perhaps plant vines to cover the institutional look. Green chain link fencing such as that used around tennis courts would be a better choice. In one setting a gazebo with seating, about 40' apart in one direction encouraged walking among the stronger ambulatory residents, while seating groups along other paths at every 20' accommodated the more frail population (Hiatt, 1979). Sometimes baffle fencing is necessary to shelter residents from wind and breezes.

In the same facility a patio, while it offered another opportunity for outside activities, was underutilized. Three possible reasons for underusage could be the heat, lack of planned activities and lack of accessibility. Suggestions for correcting these problems, while obvious, could be further strengthened by introducing large, potted plants to provide shade and adding raised flower boxes for resident participation in gardening activities.

ENTRY

The front door of a facility must be easy to open and should include a window to prevent collisions. Thresholds should be eliminated to prevent tripping and for ease in moving wheelchairs. For the frail population, automatic door openers should be considered. Sufficient pressure adjustments to establish a net opening force of less than eight pounds and time-delayed action are recommended for automatic door closers (Kiewel, Salmen, 1977).

The main lobby, or foyer, in a long-term care facility carries many of the same implications as any other entry area. The intention is to provide space for entry that is welcoming and functional. It is in the area of function that the nursing home may differ. Often the foyer becomes a gathering place for residents to "people-watch." While this is a normal and often enjoyable past-time, it is likely to intrude on the welcoming aspect of the area because of congestion. The space in the entry area in one facility served as a reception area for visitors and a waiting/watching area for residents. In a U-shaped facility the nurses station was located adjacent to the entry area and the administrator's office was where two of the wings met. The recommendation included switching the nurses station with the administrator's office. This would reduce the combined nurses station/entry congestion and bring the administrator near the front door, a better public relations location. There was also potential for the redesign of some kitchen storage space into a small lounge area directly adjacent to the foyer.

RESIDENT ROOMS

If facility redesign is to be successful, more emphasis must be placed on the design of the resident's room. Essential to this design is a chair that is comfortable, accessible and stable, floor covering that is safe and easy to maintain, window treatment that controls glare and lighting that provides adequate illumination. Beyond these basic concerns is the acute need to make this limited space "home." Issues of personalization, privacy and control are very important environmental attributes that have been addressed in another section of this publication. While adapting this environment for the age-related needs of the individual these psychological considerations must not be overlooked.

For the patient in acute care, the wall-mounted position for the television is satisfactory. For the person who is seated, either in the room chair or a wheelchair, there is danger of basal artery impingement when the head is bent back, looking upward, for an extended length of time. In the short-term care rooms in one facility, it was recommended that sets mounted high on the wall be lowered and placed on top of a built-in dresser or on a shelf.

The resident bathrooms, while serving an obvious function, rarely provide adequate age-related adaptations nor are they designed to be aesthetically pleasing. For instance, in several of these long-term care facilities, color contrast and lighting were major considerations. There was good contrast between the edge of the toilet seat and the floor in one facility, but the lighting was not adequate. In another facility the stool was the same off white color as the shiny vinyl floor. The ceramic tile in another, although in excellent condition, was all white. Colored toilet seats that contrast with the floor color, plastic mounted posters, colored towels and color coordinated grab bars were a few inexpensive suggestions that could improve both the appearance of the bathroom and the resident's level of functioning.

Another space that needed to be addressed was the area around the sink. In one facility, a shelf, paper towel and soap dispensers were not only mounted too high for the residents to reach, but the items that were stored on this shelf were more for staff use than for residents. It was recommended that all of these items be stored in an easily accessible but less conspicuous cupboard. Since many of the residents in this facility were in wheelchairs, additional suggestions included the placement of a cantilevered mirror, which tips out from the wall, above the sink so the person sitting in a wheelchair would be able to see themself. A lower towel bar and shelf should be placed on the wall beside the sink. The light fixtures should create minimal shadows and/or glare.

Color contrast is helpful in many activities of daily living. The toothbrush should contrast with the sink, the slippers with the floor, the toilet seat with the floor color. Colored towels that contrast with the walls would not only be visually helpful, but psychologically invigorating.

LOUNGES

Depending on the number of community spaces in the facility, lounges are often day rooms. If there is only one space, it is a "multipurpose" room. This concept is an enigma because the context of space changing for various functions is not congruent with our experiential background. We go to the theater for a movie, church for services and the Dairy Queen for a cone. These activities rarely occur in the same place.

Several facilities had multipurpose rooms. When one room serves several purposes, it was recommended that staff help orient residents to the particular activity by using specific words and symbols on a sign in front of and inside the room when that activity occurs. Some suggestions were: for a happy hour, use lettering and a beer mug or wine glass; for music groups, print MUSIC, with a musical note; for church services, use lettering plus the picture of a church.

Suggestions for church services to be held in the multipurpose room included: enhancement of the environment by changing banners which include religious symbols. Banners can be rolled and stored easily when not in use; a drape on a traverse roof would have panels of religious symbols and colors directly on the fabric; a self-contained pulpit unit would have storage for hymnals, Bibles, prayer books, communion items and other articles used in the services.

A large day room is a mixed blessing. The size alone has pros and cons: it accommodates large meetings, but does not promote a residential look and feel. Such a space can promote interaction among residents if these connections allow those passing by and those within the social spaces to see what is happening around them with minimal commitment. At least two variables must exist to foster interaction: for the person not experiencing dementia, an activity must be taking place, and the resident must have adequate vision to determine there are others in the space. Studies show that too much visual connection can cause an underutilization of some areas, however, because individuals dislike the feeling that others are watching their movements (Howell, 1980).

For instance, family visits require some visual privacy. In one facility, the placement of dividers was recommended in part of the day room to provide limited visibility for part of the lounge/day room space. Because of their acoustical properties, dividers, used in open office systems, could be adapted for the nursing home.

In another facility, furniture, arranged in several conversational groupings to promote social interaction was suggested. These arrangements should have lounge chairs at right angles to one another with a table holding a very stable table lamp in between (Sommer, 1970). In extreme cases a wood-based lamp could be bolted to the bottom of the table.

Considering the wheelchair/ambulatory ratio, places should be left for wheelchairs. The activities department in one facility gave excellent input on the flexibility needed for the lounge space. This staff should be consulted concerning space utilization particularly, for a large group.

In one nursing home, the staff felt some rocking chairs were appropriate for the area. Because of its stability, the chair that was recommended was a glider design. In this particular facility the other lounge chairs should be in keeping with the residential tone of the room. All chairs should be selected using the criteria on chairs included in the section dealing with chair design.

One facility had a large, new television set in the lounge. However, it was not located at the best height. It was recommended that it be raised and put into the built-in cabinet available. The eye level of the seated elderly tall male is 48.6" and the small female is 37.4", making the average eye level approximately 43" (Panero & Zelnik, 1979). Elderly upward gaze has lowered and, due to osteoporosis or reduced mobility of the neck, often there is about five degrees of forward tilt to the head. Considering these figures and based on viewing the television from a distance of ten to twelve feet, the center of the screen should be placed approximately 32" above the floor. Some chairs should be arranged in this viewing area, but space needs to be left for persons in wheelchairs.

CHAPEL

In one facility the major problem in the chapel was the carpeting near the front of the sanctuary. Older residents who wished to be involved in services by reading, could not get up and down the carpeted area to the lectern. It was suggested that a wooden hand-rail, in keeping with the serene, grand nature of the space, be placed at the corner of the platform steps. New carpet, in a color to match banners, with a strip of lighter color woven directly to define the edge of the step, would satisfy aesthetic and safety factors. An alternative suggestion was to include an indirect strip of lighting along these steps.

It was recommended that kneeling benches contrast in color with the floor surface and lighting be increased. Two other considerations were wheelchair accessibility and hearing amplification devices to combat acoustical problems.

DINING ROOM

In one facility, a large open area in the dining room created an institutional appearance. This effect was heightened by the addition of a bulletin board and activity calendar and a brick end wall. The suggestion for this space was to place quilts, made by a local quilter, as wall hangings on the brick wall and another wall in the dining room and to move the activity calendar to a lighted corridor wall next to the activity area. The residents would be more apt to read it there.

Direct glare was a major issue in this dining room as the light from the window reflects off the highly polished vinyl floor tile. To reduce direct glare, the recommendation included the installation of vertical blinds. The day room and dining room share the same window so the vertical blinds would also be utilized for the dayroom.

Floor covering that has little or no glare should be installed in both areas. Carpet was discussed for the lounge space but because of food spillage and staining, the staff preferred a hard surface floor for the dining space. Vinyl bonded wood that creates a minimum of indirect glare was recommended for the dining room. This type of flooring has been used quite successfully in long-term care facilities. It provides a warmth and residential feel that does not exist with vinyl. The initial cost would be higher than vinyl composition tile, but life cycle cost is less because of durability and ease of maintenance. No waxing is necessary.

NURSES STATION

The input of the nursing staff, must be considered for design details that meet their needs. Recommendations focused on how the design of a nurses station affected the behavior of the residents and modifications or adaptations which might improve that functioning.

The counter in several of these facilities was 45″ to 48″. Since the eye level of older persons in wheelchairs will be less than that, it is often difficult for the resident to have eye contact with the nurse behind the counter unless one of them stands up, usually the nurse. Because the resident may not see or hear well, he/she will move into the entrance to the nurses station which causes additional congestion. It was recommended part of the counter be lowered to desk height to eliminate some of this behavior. If charting is done in this area, part of the counter should be left at the original height.

To de-emphasize the medical and institutional nature of a nursing home, ways need to be devised to remove the nurses station as the hub of activity. Terminology can also have an impact. When the counter is lowered to desk height, it should be referred to as the nurses desk rather than the more institutional term "station."

Design needs to be considered that will allow residents to watch activity by the nurses station less obtrusively and solve congestion problems which occur when wheelchairs block the entrance to the station. Arrangements for porch-type lounge spaces across from the nurses desk were recommended for one facility.

Design solutions for the nursing station in another nursing home involved a choice between several architectural solutions. The original space was too large and the staff felt the space could be better utilized. The staff requested a space utilization study for design interventions contingent upon construction restraints.

In this facility there was a need for a charting room and a medications room, but staff felt they could be combined into a smaller space. A circular, revolving chart rack would take up less room and allow the two functions to take place in one area. Redesign was needed to meet the code requirements. In the case of the medication room, Minnesota code requires "a quiet, convenient area, separated from all soiled activities shall contain a work counter, a sink with institutional fittings, a single-service towel dispenser, a refrigerator for medications with a reliable thermometer, and medicine and narcotics cabinet" (4660.1700 MN Rules, 1987, pg. 95-96). The redesigned space would provide a more functional lounge area where residents could congregate without causing congestion at the nurses station.

One 100-bed facility, built 18 years ago as an extension of a hospital, was designed with a central nurses station at the core of five color-coded wings. One long wing connects the nursing home to the hospital and contains the activity/dining room, chapel and the physical and occupational therapy areas. The remaining wings are assigned to residents according to their degrees of independence. The very large central nurses station takes up the entire middle space of the core area. Staff had determined that this amount of space for the nurses station was no longer necessary. Several design solutions were presented, all of which reduced the size of the nurses station and allowed more space for resident activity.

When the nurses station is reduced in size a study needs to be conducted to determine the affect upon the resident behavior. One hypothesis would be that when the nurses station is no longer the "hub of activity" congestion caused by the residents would decrease.

BATHING/TUB ROOM

Codes provide guidelines for existing construction of central bathing areas. Bathing areas with more than one fixture should have privacy curtains and/or wall dividers. Bathtubs and showers should have a nonslip floor surface. Rubberized flooring is recommended in these areas. If there is a toilet in the area, it must be provided with privacy curtains or small partitions and grab bars on both sides of the toilet. New construction codes are more detailed. Minnesota code requires at least one bathtub or shower area, designed for assisted bathing. Codes include specific instructions for size of shower stalls and tubs. Grab bars, folding shower seats, flexible hose hand-held showers, recessed soap holders without handles are specified (Minn. Health Dept., 1987). Many of these items can be color coordinated and incorporated into existing rooms to provide aesthetic appeal as well as safety and dignity.

Bath time is often traumatic for both staff and residents. This is particularly true when the resident must be undressed in their rooms and then transported down the corridor to a tub room. Recommendations to the facilities, that followed this procedure, were to try and design a space in the tub room to undress and dress the resident.

In one nursing home, one public rest room could be eliminated, the wall removed and a dressing space designed adjacent to the tub. In another facility, a dressing space was conceivable by taking footage from an adjoining room. Those persons who must be conveyed undressed through the corridors could be provided with soft terry robes rather than being drapped with a bath blanket. Redesigning the tub room to make it more inviting by adding colored towels, more attractive wallcover, lighting and plants may help reduce bath time trauma but attention to privacy and dignity issues must be the first consideration.

BARBER/BEAUTY SHOP

Some of the same concerns that exist for elderly persons who watch television with an extended head position apply to the person in a beauty shop chair. The beauty shop chair should allow the entire back to be tipped back with the feet and legs of the resident elevated as his/her hair is shampooed. For the resident who cannot be transferred into a beauty shop chair, the facility should have at least one wheelchair with a reclining back.

DESIGN CONSIDERATIONS FOR DEMENTIA UNITS

In order to address the needs of the resident with dementia many facilites are designing separate wings that can accommodate the ambulatory, confused person. Principle considerations when planning for this old, expanding group are safety and space.

As facilities have learned to cope with their wandering, disoriented residents many innovative solutions have been tried. A few ideas are included here and elsewhere in this publication.

Safety

The person who wanders has gained the most attention, albeit negative, when administrators and planners are considering the needs of residents with dementia. Although these persons are clearly an enormous legal and administrative burden, there are some comforting findings with respect to environmental adaptations.

The best solutions to the problem of wandering make it difficult for the resident to locate the exit. Where codes will allow, elevator buttons can be covered with pictures or signs. A study by Namazi et al. (1989) examined different visual barriers for doors to reduce patient exits. The most successful intervention was the placement of a cloth panel over the doorknob. Plants, gates, screens or other barriers can be placed in corridors to confine residents to a wing or a section of the facility.

Windows must be secured so residents can not climb out. Caulkins (1988) has warned against certain types of bedrails. The confused person may get their feet caught in them. If railings are essential select a type that does not fold down to the floor.

Since the person with Alzheimer's disease often has poor judgement, safety concerns such as electrical cords, hot coffee urns and room heaters need to be considered, much as they might be with young children. The environment should not be sterile in appearance but does need to be as uncomplicated as practical by removing precious decorative items and securing lamps or furniture, all issues that have been addressed in this publication.

Space

Persons with mental impairment often find it difficult to sit for long periods of time or, in some instances, to sit at all with restlessness pervading most activities. The reasons for the need to pace are unclear although it is not a universal trait of the person with dementia. Nevertheless, facilities have found it helpful to have a large area, either out of doors (more appropriate in the sunbelt states) or as an extension of the wing where the dementia residents live. This could be a corridor, winterized sun room, or designated lounge away from the dining or day room where others may be sitting. Several facilities have created a "race track" design in which the pacer can follow an endless visual path created by the carpet (Caulkins, 1988). If space does not allow for an actual pathway, some facilities have had success by creating a visual line with the carpet which the pacers seem to follow. Not surprisingly, the pacing resident can be upsetting to other residents who are trying to reduce their own confusion and adjust to an unfamiliar environment.

These are just a few suggestions that have been successful. The environmental needs of the person with dementia are only beginning to be addressed by designers and planners. As we gain experience serving these residents our solutions will be more appropriate to meet their needs.

In the future, special design considerations for residents with senile dementia will benefit from studies of buildings that respond to their profound needs. With Alzheimer's Disease predicted to be of epidemic proportions in the next century, any redesign of present long-term care facilities must incorporate recommendations that are functional and practical for the dementia population.

CONCLUSION

The Health Care Finance Administration has placed a strong emphasis on "environmental quality" in the new Medicaid and Medicare requirements which will become effective in 1990 (Erickson, 1989). As renewed focus is placed upon the physical environment, the need to evaluate and redesign not only the structure but the thinking of the way that space is utilized must be a major consideration.

The application of research that provides insight into the environmental needs of the older person will provide us with new approaches to maximize their function. The application, by manufacturers, of new materials and the development of products that meet the needs of the older population will provide us with tangible ways to implement those approaches. Creating the utmost in environmental quality for the older person is more than just a pleasant sounding phrase, it is a doable concept whose time has come.

Appendix

GUIDELINES FOR SELECTING LANDMARKS AND SIGNAGE

1. LANDMARKS

A. *Wall Covering*

The pattern, texture and/or color of the wall covering is a subtle method of orientation and sets the background for landmarks. The ideal corridor wall treatment is one that has definite pattern in certain areas and areas that are plain or with minimal design. These open areas provide a spot for distinctive landmarks.

B. *Matting*

Matting can add a great deal in the way of contrast to a picture. A light mat between a dark tone picture and a darker wall, or vice versa, is more apparent for the resident with reduced vision. For the person with very limited vision, matting of intense contrast will produce a landmark even if the individual is unable to see the detail in the picture.

C. *Framing*

Framing on pictures should have rounded corners and no sharp edges. Non-glare 1/16th" glass should be used. If glass is thicker, it causes distortion of the image.

D. *Requirements*

All landmarks must be made of material that is easy to clean and is fire retardant.

E. *Principles for Selection*

There are five basic principles for the selection of art work that will be used for landmarks. These considerations are: contrast of light and dark, use of color, size of subject matter, recognizable themes, and content that relates to the background of the residents.

1. *Contrast of Light and Dark:*

As visual acuity decreases for the elderly the need for marked contrast increases. For signs, white on black provides the most contrast (Cooper, 1986). Other detail should be considered with the same eye to distinct differences in shades and tints.

Intense colors used adjacent to each other cause the eye to fatigue. However, these strong color combinations are orienting. Therefore, as cues, there are places where these bold contrasts are valuable. If the same colors were selected for a lounge they might not be appropriate.

2. *Use of Color:*
   A wide range of colors can be chosen. The major concern with most pictures is that many shades of a color are used and thus the entire picture becomes muted. Because of yellowing of the lens of the eye, blues and greens adjacent to each other will be difficult for the older person to discern. Sharp bright color contrasts are most pleasing. More research needs to be done into the psychology of color and the elderly. Advocating or avoiding certain colors because of their "effect" on an older person is not well documented.

3. *Size of Subject:*
   Main subject matter should be discernable at twenty feet (Hiatt, 1980). However, if subject matter is too large, i.e., a graphic or mural, because of the older person's reduction in peripheral vision, some detail will be outside the visual field.

4. *Theme of picture:*
   Design should be simple, clear and realistic. If only a bold color or accent is desired, abstract painting may be appropriate. However, for older persons the subject matter that is most appreciated is that which closely resembles reality.

5. *Background of the Residents:*
   The resident should be able to relate to the theme of the picture. Pictures of the city are not as appropriate in a rural facility or desert scenes in a facility in northern states. Universal favorites seem to be children, flowers, ships, mountain and, probably due to our agrarian past, farm scenes.

F. *Textured Wall Hangings*

1. *Fabric Graphics*
   There are some excellent fabric graphics available which have pleasing distinct color combinations and minimal detail. Fabric graphics can be incorporated with wall covering to set a definite theme in a corridor.

Fabric graphics can be found in almost any price range. The two-dimensional type are relatively inexpensive. Soft sculptures and three-dimensional raised designs cost considerably more. The advantages of the latter are that they add tactile input and provided redundant cueing (Pastalan, 1973) in these spaces.

2. *Quilts*

Quilts can be utilized very effectively. They can be designed to coordinate with a specific color scheme and because of their significance as a part of American folk art, are important.

3. *Wall Hangings*

There are a variety of commercial wall hangings on the market. These are usually composed of yarns of various thicknesses and the designs tend to be more abstract. This type of wall hanging does provide excellent texture.

4. *Carpet*

Pictorial designs have been developed using carpet of different colors and at varying heights.

5. *Wood Carvings*

Wood carvings highlighted with colored stains make excellent landmarks.

2. SIGNS

Whereas landmarks are specific cues, signage is designed to guide a person through a designated space to a specific spot. Signs may become landmarks. This may occur because the sign dominates the space or it may be specifically planned by the staff.

A. *Location*

Considerations for the location of signs should include: the smaller stature of the older person, a slight forward tilt in their standing posture, reduced vision and decreased upward gaze. Because of these concerns, sign placement should be no higher than 4 1/2 feet above the floor and as low as 2 inches above the handrail. Signs should be mounted on the wall on the side which the door opens.

B. *Types*

Several different types of signs are available. Signs with surface applied vinyl letters and/or numbers often do not last because these digits can be scraped off. Recessed and raised numerals add helpful tactile cues. On raised digits dirt collects and creates problems for housekeeping. The raised letters may also create a slight shadow and make the sign harder to read. Signs on which the printing is reverse silkscreened (from the back) are the easiest to maintain. A 1/16th inch non-glare plastic should overlay these signs. If the plastic is thicker than 1/16th inch a shadow will be created which can be visually disorienting.

C. *Requirements*
There are different requirements and arrangements for resident room signs. The sign must contain the room number and the resident's name. The number should be 2″ in height and the resident's name 5/8″ to 3/4″ each in height. Size of letters may be dependent on the type of lettering system the facility uses.

D. *Signs for Dementia*
For residents with dementia, ideally the sign should contain a space where some type of orienting symbol or color can be affixed with double sided tape. Signs incorporating pictures or photographs, of the individual engaged in some meaningful activity or persons and places that have special meaning to the resident, have been used successfully. Current photographs may not have meaning for the resident.

SPOT REMOVAL MAINTENANCE

The single most difficult problem in carpet maintenance is that of stains, usually the result of spills. Hospitals, child care centers, and recuperation facilities are most often cited as illustrations; but office buildings and other public buildings are also plagued with an astonishing range of staining problems, from tracked-in grease and wax to beverage and chemical stains. All of these require a well planned and conscientiously followed spotting program.

Immediate action following a spill can work wonders on stains that, after becoming dry might be extremely difficult, if not impossible, to completely remove. Do not depend on periodic shampooing to remove stains. Proper identification is important to successful stain removal. Since many stains, such as coffee with cream, are both water and grease base, at least two agents are often required. Handy spotting kits with stain analyzer and removal guides are retailed widely and can be quite effective if used properly. Be patient and avoid overwetting the carpet, which can spread the stain or cause bleeding from binders or from jute backing. Repeated applications are often necessary to remove heavy concentrated spills. The stain will continue reappearing after drying as it is wicked up from the base of the pile until the substance has been completely removed. Large stains dissolved in detergent or water can often be effectively and quickly taken up with a wet vacuum, minimizing spreading.

General Procedures for Spot Removal

1. Absorb wet spills with tissue, white cloth or paper towels, or a clean sponge. A weighted pad of tissue left in place for a short time is often very effective.
2. Determine composition of stain and follow procedure recommended on the chart provided. Stains of unknown composition should be treated first with a volatile solvent, followed by other agents as required. If uncertain about effect of an agent on carpet fiber or dye, test first on an inconspicuous area. Apply a small amount, press an absorbent tissue to the stain for ten seconds, and see if there is any dye transfer or fiber damage.
3. Work from outside to center to prevent spread of the stain or formation of a ring. Avoid rubbing, which only spreads stain and distorts the pile. Do not rush the job, as many stains require time to respond.
4. If the stain is hard or crusty, tap it with a brush to work the cleaning agent into the pile and help break up the staining material.
5. Repeat applications of small amounts of agent and absorption of dissolved material until the stain is satisfactorily removed.
6. Use a fan or weighted tissues to dry the cleaned area. Rapid evaporation or absorption of the cleaning agent is desirable to prevent wetting through to the backing and possible jute staining.

Spot Removal Supplies

If the spot removal is included in an outside cleaning service contract, the cleaning agents and equipment will normally be supplied by the service company. If the spot removal is to be done by the in-house custodial staff it is important that adequate supplies of materials are available.

Suggested Supplies:

- Abundance of absorbent white cloth or towels for blotting.
- Sponges for blotting.
- Spatulas (tongue depressors will do) for mild scraping and removal of excess sudsy detergent.
- Large carry tray or cart.
- Wet vacuum or portable hot water extraction unit for large spills.
- Small, soft hand spotting brushes.

- Trigger spray bottles-1 quart size.
- Squeeze bottles-1 pint size.

Suggested Spotting Agents:

The following agents can be made up from easily obtained products by the custodial staff as follows:

- Detergent solution — 1 tablespoon of dry powder household detergent (without bleach) per pint of water. White vinegar solution — 50% water/50% vinegar.
- Ammonia solution — 2 tablespoons of ammonia in 1/2 cup (4 oz.) water — make stronger as needed.
- Plain water — for rinsing.
- Alcohol — regular rubbing or denatured — use as is.
- Dry cleaning fluid — a common non-flammable brand, used according to manufacturer's directions.

The agents listed below can usually be obtained from janitor and custodial supply companies:

- Paint, Oil and Grease Remover — referred to as P.O.G.
- Picrin — a volatile dry clean spotter. Perchlorethylene-dry cleaner solvent.
- Amyl Acetate — a common drugstore brand or nail polish remover without lanolin.
- Hydrofluoric Acid — rust stains are most easily removed with hydrofluoric acid. However, this is a dangerous chemical and should be handled only by trained personnel. It can be purchased from suppliers to service companies at 5% or 10% concentration and should be used in this form without further dilution.
- Oxalic Acid — this agent is less dangerous than hydrofluoric acid for removing rust stains and a little less effective. Adequate rinsing and blotting is necessary after the stain disappears to remove any residual crystals.

Spray Preparations:

There are many spray preparations and other labeled all-purpose spot removal agents on the market with varying degrees of effectiveness. Many leave a residue on the carpet that can readily attract soil and also affect carpet color. Before using, these preparations should be applied and blotted for color transfer on a small inconspicuous area of carpet and allowed to dry for a day or two and rechecked. The safest way to use these preparations is to rinse with detergent solution and plain water after using to blot up all residue possible.

Note: Cleaning agent containers should be clearly labeled.

REMOVAL PROCEDURES FOR SPECIFIC STAINS

STAIN	REMOVAL PROCEDURE
Acetone	Absorb
Alcohol, Ethyl	Absorb
Asphalt	Use volatile solvent
Beer	Absorb, use detergent, water, acetic acid
Berry Stain	Absorb, use detergent/ammonia (3-6% solution), water
Blood (wet)	Absorb, use detergent/ammonia (3-6% solution), hydrogen peroxide
Blood (dried)	Scrape, use warm detergent/ammonia (3-6% solution), water, or use chemical enzyme
Bleach	Use detergent, water
Butter	Spoon, use volatile solution
Calcium Chloride-powder	Vacuum, use detergent, water
Calcium Chloride 10%	Absorb, use detergent, water
Carbon Black	Vacuum, use detergent, water, and volatile solvent
Chewing Gum	Freeze with Chemspec Chewing Gum Remover in aerosol can, shatter and vacuum, or use volatile solvent
Chocolate	Absorb, use detergent/ammonia (3-6% solution), water
Clay (red)	Vacuum, use detergent, water, acetic acid

Coffee (black)	Absorb, use detergent, water, acetic acid
Coffee (sugar & cream)	Absorb, use detergent, water, acetic acid, volatile solvent
Cola Drink	Absorb, use detergent, water
Crayon (red)	Use paint remover, volatile solvent
Creme de Menthe	Absorb, use detergent/ammonia (3-6% solution), water
Crepe Paper Dye	Use detergent/ammonia (3-6% solution), water
Duco Cement	Use paint remover, volatile solvent
Egg (raw)	Spoon and absorb, use detergent, water
Ether	Absorb, use detergent, water
Food Color	Absorb, use detergent/ammonia (3-6% solution), water
Furniture Dye	Absorb, use paint remover, volatile solvent, alcohol, detergent/ammonia (3-6% solution), water
Gentian Violet	Use alcohol, detergent, water
Grape Juice	Absorb, use detergent/ammonia (3-6% solution), water
Gravy	Absorb, use detergent, water
Grease (car)	Use volatile solvent
Ice Cream	Spoon and absorb, use detergent water
Ink (washable)	Use detergent/ammonia (3-6% solution), water, acetic acid
Ink (ball point)	Use paint remover, volatile solvent, detergent, water
Ink (India)	Absorb, use paint remover, volatile solvent, detergent, water
Ink (permanent)	Absorb, use paint remover, volatile solvent, detergent, water

Iodine	Absorb, use alcohol, potassium iodide, sodium thiosulfate, sodium hypochlorite, detergent, water
Iron Rust	Vacuum, use hydrofluoric acid, water
Lacquer	Absorb, use paint remover, methylene, chloride, detergent, water
Linseed Oil	Absorb, use volatile solvent
Lipstick	Use paint remover, volatile solvent
"Lysol"	Use paint remover, volatile solvent, detergent, water
Mascara	Use paint remover, volatile solvent, detergent, water
"Merthiolate"	Absorb, use alcohol, detergent/ ammonia (3-6% solution), water
Milk	Absorb, use detergent, water
Mucilage	Absorb, use detergent/ammonia (3-6% solution), water
Mustard	Spoon and absorb, use detergent, acetic acid, hydrofluoric acid, water
Nail Polish	Absorb, use amyl acetate, volatile solvent
Oil	Use volatile solvent
Orange Drink	Absorb, use detergent/ammonia (3-6% solution), water
Paint (oil base)	Spoon and absorb, use paint remover, methylene chloride, detergent, water
Paint (water base)	Spoon and absorb, use paint remover, methylene chloride, detergent, water
Phenol 1%	Use detergent, water
Rubber Cement	Spoon and absorb, use paint remover, volatile solvent

Shoe Polish (paste or liquid)	Absorb with heated iron into towel, use paint remover, volatile solvent, detergent, water
Shoe Polish (liquid)	Absorb, use paint remover, volatile solvent, detergent, water
Tea	Absorb, use detergent, water
Tomato Juice	Absorb, use detergent, water
Urine	Absorb, use detergent, water, acetic acid
Vesphene	Absorb, use detergent, water
Vomit	Spoon and absorb, use warm detergent, water, acetic acid and/or enzyme
Water colors	Absorb, use detergent/ammonia (3-6% solution), water
Wax (candle)	Absorb with heated iron into towel, use volatile solvent (use synthetic setting on iron)
Wescodyne	Absorb, use alcohol, potassium iodine, sodium thiosulfate, sodium hypochlorite, detergent, water
Wine	Absorb, use detergent/ammonia (3-6% solution), water, acetic acid
Zephiran, Tinct.	Absorb, use detergent, water

Permission to reprint this information has been granted by:

BASF Corporation
Fibers Division
Williamsburg, VA 23187

"The information contained herein is the best that we have available to us on the subject. However, BASF Fibers makes no guarantee of results or assumes no responsibility whatsoever in connection with its use, nor is any license granted hereby. Neither is anything herein intended as a recommendation to infringe any patent" (BASF Corporation).

1. What devices and/or interventions did you receive?

2. Which items have you used?

3. If there were items you did not use, what were the reasons you did not use them?

4. What are some less desirable aspects about the device(s)? i.e. the numbers on the phone are not large enough, etc.

5. What changes would you make in the design(s)? i.e. larger numbers on the phone, more space between numbers for easier dialing, etc.

6. Did the device(s) allow you to feel safe?

7. Did the device(s) allow you to do a task(s) more easily?

8. Now that you know the effectiveness of the devices you were provided, would you have been willing to purchase them yourself?

___Yes. Which ones?_____
_____
_____

___No.   Because
          a. __ Price
          b. __ Difficult to operate
          c. __ Difficult to install
          d. __ Difficult to obtain
          e. __ Didn't need
          f. __ Other_____

9. Are there any tasks which you would like to do more easily? Explain.

10. Additional Comments

NOTE: If self-administered, questionnaire should be printed in large type.

Device and/or Intervention Satisfaction Questionnaire

REFERENCES

Accident Facts (1985) *National Hospital Discharge Survey, Stock No. 044-218* Washington D.C.: US Public Health Service.

Altman I (1974) Privacy: A conceptual analysis, In D. Carson (ed.) *EDRA 5: Man-Environment interactions: Evaluations and Application* Milwaukee, WI: Environmental Design Research Association.

AOTA (1983) *Architectural Barriers/OT's Consulting to Architects* Rockville, MD: American Occupational Therapy Association.

Archea JC (1985) Environmental Factors Associated with Stair Accidents by the Elderly, *Clinics in Geriatric Medicine*, 1(3): 555-569.

Asher JK (1977) Toward a safer design for stairs, *Job Safety and Health* 5:27-32.

Azar GJ & Lawton AH (1964) Gait and Stepping as Factors in the Frequent Falls of Elderly Women, *Gerontologist*; 4(2): 83-84, 103.

Baker SP & Harvey AH (1985) Fall Injuries in the Elderly *Clinics in Geriatric Medicine*, 1(3), 501-508.

Bell LW (1989) Involuntary relocation of the elderly: recovery following a fire disaster *Unpublished Masters, Thesis* Univ. of Minn.

Bexton WH, Heron W & Scott TH (1954) Effects of Decreased Variation in the Sensory Environment *Canadian Journal of Psychology* 8:70-76.

Birren J & Schaie K (1977) *Handbook of the Psychology of Aging* New York: Van Nostrand Reinhold Co.

Bostrom JA, Mace RL & Long M (1987) *Adaptable Housing*, Raleigh, NC: Barrier Free Environments, Inc.

Bowersox J (1979) Architectural and Interior Design *Long Term Care of the Aging: A Socially Responsible Approach*, ed. Lois J. Wasser, Washington, D.C., American Assoc. of Homes for the Aging.

Brink CA & Wells TJ (1986) Environmental Support for Geriatric Incontinence *Clinics in Geriatric Medicine* 2(4):829-840, November.

Busse E (1978) How Mind, Body and Environment Influence Nutrition in the Elderly *Postgraduate Medicine* 63(3):118-125, March.

Calkins MP (1988) *Design for Dementia* Owings Mills, MD: National health Publishing.

Campbell AJ, Reinken J, Allan BC & Martinez GS (1981) Falls in Old Age: a Study of Frequency and Related Clinical Factors *Age and Aging* 10:264-270.

Carson DH, Archea JC, Margulis ST & Carson FE (1978) Safety on Stairs Washington D.C.: National Bureau of Standards U.S. Government Printing Office.

Carstens DY (1985) *Site Planning and Design for the Elderly* New York: Van Nostrand Reinhold Company.

Chalke H & Dewhurst J (1957) Coal Gas Poisoning: Loss of Sense of Smell as a Possible Contributing Factor with Old People *British Medical Journal* 2:1915-1917.

Christenson, B (1989) Personal conversation, October.

Christenson MA (1988) Unpublished results, Phase I of SBIR Grant.

Christenson MA & Raschko BA (1989) Environmental Cognition and Age-Related Sensory Change *Occupational Therapy Practice* 1:1 To be published in December 1989.

Colavita F (1978) *Sensory Changes in the Elderly* Springfield, IL: Charles C. Thomas.

Comalli (1965) Cognitive Functioning in a Group of 80-90 Year Old Men *Journal of Gerontology*, 20:14-17.

Comalli P (1967) Perception and Age *Gerontologist*, 7(2):73-77.

COMSIS Corp. (1988) *Product Safety and the Older Consumer*, U.S. Consumer Product Safety Commission, Washington D.C: U.S. Govn't Printing Office.

Cooper BA, Gowland C & McIntosh J (1986) The Use of Color in the Environment of the Elderly to Enhance Function *Clinics in Geriatric Medicine* 2(1)151-163.

Corso J (1971) Sensory Processes of Age Effects in Normal Adults *Journal of Gerontology* 26(1):90-105.

Cristarella MC (1977) Visual Function of the Elderly *American Journal of Occupational Therapy* 31(7):432-440, August.

Csikszenthmihalyi M & Rochberg-Halton E (1981) *The Meaning of Things: Domestic Symbols and the Self*, Cambridge: Cambridge University Press.

Devlin AS (1980) Housing for the Elderly *Environment and Behavior* 12:453-466.

Division of Injury Epidemiology and Control Center 1986 Annual Report (1987) Environmental Health: Center for Disease Control, January.

Eisdorfer C (1968) Arousal and performance: Experiments in verbal learning and a tentative theory, In G. Talland (Ed.) *Human Aging and Behavior* New York: Academic Press.

Erickson J (1989) Medicare and Medicaid: requirements for Long-Term Care Facilities *Care Perspectives* Bloomington, MN: Care Providers of Minnesota, 17-19.

Ernst & Shore (1976) *Sensitizing People to the Processes of Aging: The In-service Educator's Guide* Denton, TX: Center for Studies in Aging, School of Community Service, North Texas State University.

Finely F, Cody K & Finiz R (1969) Locomotion Patterns in Elderly Women *Archives of Physical Medicine* 50:140-146.

Finlay OE (1981) Rehabilitation Chair *Physiotherapy* 67(79):207.

Finlay OE, Bayles TB, Rosen C & Milling J (1983) Effects of chair design, age, and cognitive status on mobility *Age and Aging* 12:329-335.

Firestone IJ, Lichtman CM & Evans JR (1980) Privacy and Solidarity: Effects of Nursing Home Accommodations on Environmental Perception and Social Preferences *Int'l Journal of Aging and Human Development* 11(3)229-238.

Gilbert AN & Wysocki CJ (1987) The Smell Survey Results *National Geographic* 172(4)514-525 October.

Gray-Vickery, M. (1984) Education to Prevent Falls, *Geriatric Nursing* May/June.

Hadley, E., Radebaugh, T.S., & Suzman, R. (1985) Falls and Gait Disorders Among the Elderly, *Clinics in Geriatric Medicine*, 1(3), 497-500, August.

Hall G, Kirschling M & Todd S (1986) Sheltered Freedom: An Alzheimer's Unit in ICF *Geriatric Nursing* 132-137.

Harris C & Mayfield W (1983) *Selecting Chairs for Older and Disabled People Loughborough, England: Institute for Consumer Ergonomics*, University of Technology.

Hartigan JD (1982) The Dangerous Wheelchair *Journal of the American Geriatric Society* 30(9), 572-573.

Hasselkus B (1974) Aging and the Human Nervous System *American Journal of Occupational Therapy* 28(1)L16-21.

Hatton (1977) Aging and the Glare Problem *Journal of Gerontological Nursing* 3:38-44.

Hiatt LG (1975) Living Environments, Geriatric Wheelchairs and Older Person's Rehabilitation *Journal of Gerontological Nursing* 1(5)17-20 November/December.

Hiatt LG (1979) Architecture for the Aged: Design for Living *Inland Architect*, 6-18, 41-42, November and December.

Hiatt LG (1980) Is Poor Light Dimming the Sight of Nursing Home Patients *Nursing Homes* 32-41, October.

Hiatt LG (1984) Conveying the Substances of Images, Interior Design in Long Term Care *Contemporary Administrator* 7(4):17-18,20,22,55.

Hiatt LG (1985) Understanding the Physical Environment *Pride Institute Journal of Long Term Care* 4(2)12-22.

Hiatt LG (1987) Personal Conversation, July.

Howell S (1980) *Designing for Aging*, Cambridge, MA: MIT Press.

Howell S (1985) Home, A Source of Meaning in Elders' Lives *Generations* 58-60, Summer.

Huss AJ (1977) Touch With care or a Caring Touch *American Journal of Occupational Therapy* 31:11-18.

Ittelson WH, Proshansky HM & Rivlin LG (1970) Bedroom Size and Social Interaction of the Psychiatric Ward, *Environment and Behavior* 2:255-270.

Jordon J (1979) Designing Interiors for the Elderly *Executive Housekeeper*, 14-15, August.

Kaste G (1989) Personal conversation, October.

Kaufman JE (1981) *IES Lighting Handbook* New York: The Illuminating Engineering Society of North America.

Kennedy TE & Coppard LC (1987) The Prevention of Falls in Later Life *Danish Medical Bulletin*, Gerontology Special Supplement, No. 4.

Kenney JM, Stephens MAP & Brockmann AM (1987) Personal and Environmental Correlates of Territoriality and Use of Space *Environment and Behavior* 19(6)722-737 November.

Kern T (1986) Safety First: Modifying and Adapting the Environment for the Patient With Alzheimer's Disease Gerontology *Special Interest Section Newsletter*, Rockville, MD: American Occupational Therapy Association.

Kiernat J (1982) Environment: The hidden modality. *Physical and Occupational Therapy in Geriatrics*, 2(1):3-12.

Kiernat (1985) Environmental Aspects Affecting Health *Care of the Elderly: A Health Team Approach* Boston: Little, Brown & Co.

Kiewel H & Salem J (1977) *Accessible Architecture: An Illustrated Handbook based on Minn. Bldg. Chap. 55* Saint Paul, MN: Minnesota State Council for the Handicapped.

Koncelik JA (1976) *Designing the Open Nursing Home*. Stroudsburg, PA: Dowden, Hutchinson and Ross, Inc.

Kornzweig AL (1976) A Low-Vision Clinic at a Home for the Aged *Journal of the American Geriatric Society* 24(2):538-540.

Kramer L & Piermont M (1976) Rocking Water Beds and Auditory Stimuli to Enhance Growth of Preterm Infants *Journal of Pediatrics* 88:297-299

LaBuda D (1985) *The Gadget Book*, Glenview, IL: Scott, Foresman and Co.

Lang J, Burnette C, Molesti W & Vachon R (1974) *Designing for Human Behavior: Architecture and the Behavioral Sciences*, Stroudsburg, PA, Dowden, Hutchinson and Ross, Inc.

Lawton MP (1970) Public behavior of older people in congregate housing,

In J Archea & C Eastman (Eds.) Pittsburgh, PA: *Proceedings of the 2nd Environmental Design Research Association* 372-379.

Lawton MP & Bader J (1970) Wish for Privacy by young and old *Journal of Gerontology*, 35:48-54.

Lawton MP & Nahemow L (1973) Ecology and the aging process, In C Eisdoffer & MP Lawton (Eds.) *The psychology of adult development and aging*, Washington D.C.: American Psychological Assoc.

Lawton (1980) *Environment and Aging*, Monterey, CA. Brooks/Cole Publishing Co., 1980.

Leibowitz HW & Shupery CL (1985) Spatial Orientation Mechanisms and Their Implications for Falls, *Clinics in Geriatric Medicine*, 1(3), 571-580, August.

Liebowitz B, Lawton MP, & Waldman A, (1979) Evaluation: Designing for Confused Elderly People *American Institute of Architects Journal* 59-61, February.

Meier P (1978) Taking a New Look at Problems of the Old *Minneapolis Tribune* Sunday, November 19, 1978.

Melton LJ & Riggs BL (1985) Risk Factors for Injury After a Fall *Clinics in Geriatric Medicine* 1(3) August.

Millard PH and Smith CS (1981) personal Belongings-A positive Effect? *The Gerontologist*, 21(1)85-90.

Millenson M (1988) Healthcare in America *Modern Healthcare* 18(37):58-74.

Minnesota Dept of Health (1987) *Nursing; Boarding Homes; Physical Plants* Chapters 4638, 4655, 4660 Saint Paul, MN: Minnesota Documents Div.

Molotsky, I. (1985) Elderly get help from federal agencies on 3 fronts, *Minneapolis Star and Tribune*, April 16.

Montagu (1978) *Touching, The Human Significance of the Skin* New York: Harper and Row.

Murray M, Kory R, & Clarkson B (1969) Walking Patterns in Healthy Old Men *Journal of Gerontology* 24:169-178.

Namazi KH, Rosner TT & Calkins MP (1989) Visual Barriers to Prevent Ambulatory Alzheimer's Patients from Exiting Through an Emergency Door *The Gerontologist* 29(5):699-702.

National Safety Council (1981) *Fire! you can prevent it* Chicago, IL: National Safety Council.

Nickens H (1985) Falls in the aged: Medical and psychiatric issues in Dx approach, *Modern Medicine*, July.

Nuckolls J (1976) *Interior Lighting for Environmental Designers* New York: John Wiley & Sons.

O'Bryant SL (1983) The Subjective Value of "Home" to Older Home-owners *Journal of Housing for the Elderly*, 1(1)29-43 Spring/Summer.

Olin (1987) Wheelchair Seating for Older Adults *Gerontology Special Interest Section Newsletter* Rockville, MD: AOTA. 10:2,2-3.

Overstall PW, Exton-Smith AN, Imms FJ, & Johnson AL (1977) Falls in the elderly related to postural imbalance *British Medical Journal* 1:261-264.

Owen DH (1985) Maintaining Posture and Avoiding Tripping *Clinics in Geriatric Medicine* 1(3)581-599, August.

Panero J & Zelnik M (1979) *Human Dimension & Intrior Space* New York: Whitney Library of Design, Watson-Guptill Publications.

Parent L (1978) Effects of the Low-Stimulus Environment on Behavior *American Journal of Occupational Therapy* 32(1):19-25 January.

Parsons, M.T., & Levy J. (1987) Nursing Process in Injury Prevention, *Jour. of Gerontological Nursing*, 13(7),36-40.

Pastalan LA (1970) Privacy as an Expression of Human Territoriality, *Spatial behavior of older people* Ed: Leon A Pastalan and Daniel H Carson, Ann Arbor, MI: Univ. of Michigan.

Pastalan LA, Mautz R & Merrill J (1973) "The Stimulation of Age Related Sensory Losses: A New Approach to the Study of Environmental Barriers," *Environmental Design Research*, Vol. 1, Ann Arbor Michigan, Univ. of Mich.

Pastalan L, Cohen V, Steinfeld E, Weisman G & Windley P (1976) *Age Related Vision and Hearing Changes: an Empathic Approach* Ann Arbor, MI: Michigan Inst. of Geron., Univ. of Mich.

Pastalan LA & Polakow V (1986) Life Space Over the Life Span. *Journal of Housing for the Elderly*, 4(1):73-85.

Paulson D (1982) Personal Conversation, September.

Peppard N (1984) A Special Nursing Unit *Generations*, 9(2):62-63 Winter.

Pynoos J., Cohen, E., Lucas, C., & Davis, L. (1985) *The Home Evaluation Checklist and Resource Booklet for the Elderly*, Los Angeles: Robinson Foundation, UCLA/USC.

Rabizadeh, M. (1982) *Housing for the Elderly: A Self-help Guide*, Eugene, OR: University of Oregon Books.

Raschko, BB (1982) *Housing Interiors for the Disabled and Elderly* New York: Van Nostrand Reinhold Co.

Regnier V & Pynoos J (1987) *Housing the Aged*, New York: Elsevier Science Publishing Co., Inc.

Reznikoff SC (1979) *Specifications for Commercial Interiors* New York: Whitney Library of Design, Watson-Guptill Publications.

Richman L (1969) Sensory training for Geriatric Patients *American Journal of Occupational Therapy* 23:254-257.

Rullo G (1987) People and Home Interiors *Environment and Behavior* 19(2)250-259, March.

Saup W (1986) Lack of Autonomy in Old-Age Homes: A Stress and Coping Study *Journal of Housing for the Elderly*, 4(1)21-36, Spring.

Saxon SV & Etten MJ (1987) *Physical Change and Aging (2nd Edition)* New York: Tiresias Press, Inc.

Schwartz AN (1969) Perception of privacy among institutionalized aged *Proceedings of the 77th annual meeting of the American Psychological Association*, 4(2)727-728.

Schiffman (1975) Taste and Smell Changes of Foods During the Aging Process, Presentation, Louisville: Gerontological Society Annual Meeting.

Schultz DP (1965) *Sensory Restriction: Effects on Behavior* New York: Academic Press, Inc.

Shipley P (1980) Chair Comfort for the Elderly and Infirm *Medical Education (International) Ltd. Nursing* 20:858-860.

Sicurella VJ (1977) Color Contrast as an Aid for Visually Impaired Persons *Journal of Visual Impairment and Blindness* 72:252-257.

Snyder LH (1978) Environmental Changes for Socialization *Journal of Nursing Administration* 8(1)44-50.

Sommer R (1970) Small group ecology in institutions for the elderly, In L. A. Pastalan and D. H. Carson (eds.) *Spatial Behavior of Older People*, Ann Arbor, MI: Univ. of Michigan.

Sorock G et al. (1988) Benzodiazepine Sedatives and the Risk of Falling in a Community-Dwelling Elderly Cohort, *Archives of Internal Medicine*, 148, 2441-2444.

Stelman GE & Worringham CJ (1985) Sensorimotor Deficits Related to Postural Stability, *Clinics in Geriatric Medicine*, 1(3), 679-694.

Tate JW (1980) The Need for Personal Space in Institutions for the Elderly *Journal of Gerontological Nursing*, p. 439.

Technology and Aging in Minnesota (1989) Saint Paul, MN: Minnesota Gerontological Society.

U.S. Consumer Product Safety Commission Report. (1985) Administration on Aging, Department of Health and Human Services, Washington D.C.: U.S. Printing Office.

Vellas B, Cayla F, Bouquet H, dePemille F & Albarede JL (1987) Prospective Study of Restriction of Activity in Old People After Falls *Age and Aging* 16:189-193.

Walker T (1972) *Perception and Environmental Design* West Lafayette, IN: PDA Publishers.

Waller, JA (1978) *Falls among the Elderly: Human and Environmental Factors: Accident Annual and Prevention*, Pergamon Press, 10, 21-33.

Weidemann S, Anderson JR, Butterfield DI & O'Donnell PM (1982) Resident's Perceptions of Satisfaction and Safety *Environment and Behavior* 14(6)695-724, November.

Weissert, W.G. (1989) Seven Reasons Why It Is So Difficult to Make Community-Based Long-term Care Cost-Effective, *Journal of Health Education Administration*, 7(2), 423-433, Spring.

Westin A (1970) *Privacy and Freedom* New York: Atheneum Press.

Wheeler J, Woodward C, Ucovitch RL, Perry J & Walker, JM (1985) Rising from a Chair: Influence of Age and Chair design *Physical Therapy* 65(1)22-26.

Willmott M (1986) The Effect of Vinyl Floor Surface and Carpeted Floor Surface upon Walking in Elderly Hospital In-patients *Age and Aging* 15:119-120.

Windley P and Scheidt R (1980) Person-environment dialectics: Implications for competent functioning in old age. In L. Poon (ed.) *Aging in the 1980's*. Washington, D.C.: American Psychological Association.

Wolfson, LI, Whipple, R, Amerman, P, Kaplan, J, & Kleinberg, A (1985) Gait and Balance in the Elderly, *Clinics in Geriatric Medicine*, 1(3), August.

Wolanin MO & Fraelich Phillips LR (1981) *Confusion, Prevention and Care* Saint Louis: C.V. Mosby Co.

RELATED READING

American Institute of Architects, *Design for Aging: An Architect's Guide*, Washington D. C., American Institute of Architecture Press, 1985.

Aranyi L & Goldman L *Design of Long-Term Care Facilities* New York: Van Nostrand Rheinhold Co., 1980.

Azar G & Lawton, L, Gait an Stepping as Factors in the Frequent Falls of Elderly Women *The Gerontologist* 83-84,103.

Berger E (1985) The Institutionalization of the Patient's with Alzheimer's Disease *Nursing Homes* 34(6):22-29.

Campbell A, Reinken J, Allan B, Martinez G, (1981) Falls in Old Age: A Study of Frequency and Related Clinical Factors, *Age and Ageing* 264-270.

Carroll K (1978) *The Nursing Home Environment*, Minneapolis, Minnesota, Human Development in Aging Project, Ebenezer Center for Aging and Human Development.

Christenson MA (1988) Adaptations of the Physical Environment to Compensate for the Sensory Changes of Aging, *Creative Long Term Care 2nd Edition* Ed. Ken Gordon and Ruth Stryker Gordon, Springfield, IL: Charles C Thomas.

Coons D (1985) Alive and Well at Wesley Hall *Journal of Long Term Care*, Woodbridge, Ontario, 21(2).

Cooper BA (1985) A Model for Implementing Color Contrast in the Environment *The American Journal of Occupational Therapy* 39(4).

Crocker M, & Krals S (1979) An Evaluation of Nursing Home Furnishings By Occupants and Their Families, *Housing and Society* 6(2):112-119.

Delong A (1978) The Micro-Spatial Structure of the Older Person: Implications of Planning the Social and Spatial Environment, *Spatial Behavior of Older People*, Ann Arbor, Michigan, University of Michigan Press.

Drown S (1980) Effective Use of Outdoor Space for Nursing Homes: A Case Study in Progress, *Ross Timesaver* 3(1).

Finely F, Cody K & Finiz R (1969) Locomotion patterns in elderly women *Archives of Physical Medicine* 50:140-146.

Green K (1985) Design for Aging, *Architectural Technology*, 34-41, Summer.

Hanley I (1981) The Use of Signposts and Active Training to Modify Ward Disorientation in Elderly Patients, *Jour of Behavior Therapy and Exp Psychiatry* 12(3):241-247.

Hiatt LG (1981) The Color and Use of Color in Environments for Older People *Nursing Homes* 30(3):18-22.

Hiatt LG (1980) Disorientation is More than a State of Mind *Nursing Homes*, 291(4):30-36.

Hiatt LG (1980) Moving Outside and Making It a Meaningful Experience *Nursing Homes* 34-39 May/June

Hiatt LG (1982) The Importance of the Physical Environment, *Nursing Homes* 2-9.

Hiatt LG (1985) Questioning Methods of Restraining and Immobilizing Older People: Reflections from a Study on Wandering, *EDRA/16 Proceedings* 210-215, June.

Kenshalo D (1979) Changes in the Vestibular and Somesthetic Systems as a Function of Age, *Aging*, 10:269-282 New York: Raven Press.

Kromm D and Kroom YN (1985) A Nursing Unit Designed for Alzheimer's Disease Patients at Newton Presbyterian Manor, *Nursing Homes*, 34:30-31.

Lawton, MP (1970) Ecology and Aging, *Spatial Behavior of Older People*, Ed. Leon Pastalan and Daniel Carson, Ann Arbor, MI, University of Michigan.

McCorkle R (1974) Effect of Touch on Seriously Ill Patients, *Nursing Research* 23(2):125-132.

Miller, DB and Goldman L (1984) Selecting Paintings for the Nursing Home: What do Patients Prefer *Nursing Homes* 12-16.

Miller DB Goldman L and Woodman S (1985) Interior Design Preferences of Residents, Families, and Staff in Two Nursing Homes, *Journal of Long-Term Care Administrators*, 13:(3)85-89.

Pastalan L and Carson D (1984) *Spatial Behavior of Older People*, Ann Arbor, University of Michigan Press.

Pentacost R (1984) Designing for the Aging, Subtleties and Guidelines *Contemporary Administrator*, July.

Regnier V (1985) Using Outdoor Space More Effectively, *Generations*, 9(3):22-24.

Rice C, Talbott J & Stern D (1980) Effects of Environmental Agents on Social Behavior of Patients in a Hospital Dining Room, *Hospital and Community Psychiatry* 31(2):128-130.

Samton P (1974) Designing Health Care Facilities for the Elderly *American Health Care Association Journal* 33-36, July.

Tate JW (1980) The Need for Personal Space in Institutions for the Elderly *Journal of Gerontological Nursing* 6(8):439-448.

Tillock E (1979) The Humane Environment in Nursing Home Care *Nursing Homes* 22-24, May/June.

Windom, C (1982) Humanizing the Nursing Home Environment, *Nursing Homes* 32-34, January/February.